I Table of contents

I Preface

The "AO Handbook of Musculoskeletal Outcomes Measures and Instruments" is the result of a shared vision by numerous researchers and clinicians to develop a common vocabulary by which to express and share ideas regarding musculoskeletal outcomes. More than just a summary of the outcomes instruments, this book is intended to provide a solid foundation from which to advance orthopedic science.

Our intent was to identify the most commonly used musculoskeletal outcomes instruments reported in the literature (ie, those instruments which have a history of consistent use). We then proceeded to organize them first by anatomic region and then by instrument type (ie, "patient reported" or "clinician based"). Outcomes instruments that reported a single measure or score based on one physiologic outcome (ie, range of motion or radiological findings) were not included in this book.

In addition, we included the most commonly reported generic health-related quality of life instruments in the musculoskeletal literature: the Short Form 36 health survey questionnaire (SF-36), the Nottingham Health Profile (NHP), and the Musculoskeletal Function Assessment (MFA).

Our approach to identifying musculoskeletal outcomes instruments was detailed and exhaustive. We began our process by searching all of MEDLINE® to identify as many possible references in the literature containing musculoskeletal outcomes instruments. No limits were placed on the date of publication because some outcomes instruments developed several decades ago are still being used today (eg, Merle D'Aubigne-Postel hip score 1954).

Additional outcomes instruments were identified by reviewing the text and bibliographies of full-text articles and by using generic Internet search engines (eg, Google™). A list of outcomes instruments per body area was compiled and built upon throughout the search process. From this list, we first sought to locate the original article, then *all* studies in the literature that evaluated the instrument's *reliability* (reproducibility and internal consistency), *validity* (content, criterion, and construct), and *responsiveness*. Despite this challenge, in the end we feel confident that the most common musculoskeletal patient reported outcomes (PRO) and clinician based outcomes (CBO) were adequately identified in the literature.

Each instrument was reviewed and summarized with respect to four major categories:

1 Content

- Type
- Scale
- Interpretation

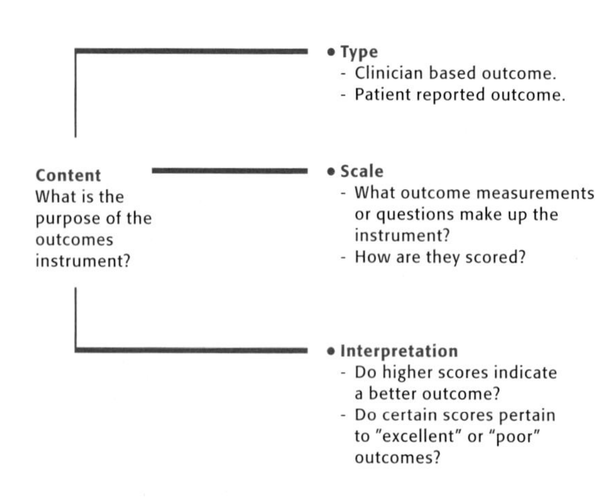

2. Methodology

- Validity
  - Construct
  - Content
  - Criterion
- Reliability
  - Internal consistency
  - Reproducibility
- Responsiveness

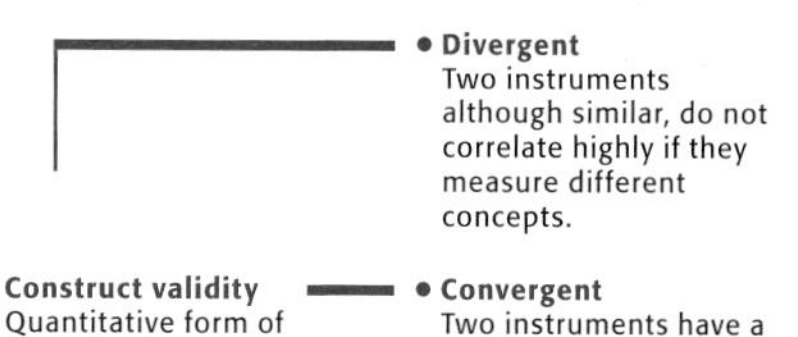

- **Divergent**
  Two instruments although similar, do not correlate highly if they measure different concepts.

- **Construct validity**
  Quantitative form of assessing instrument validity.

- **Convergent**
  Two instruments have a high correlation with each other.

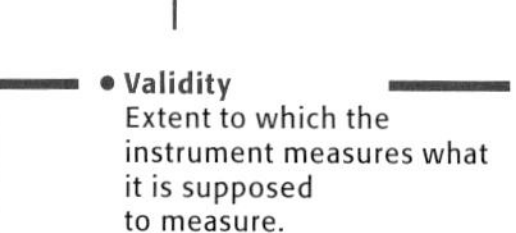

- **Validity**
  Extent to which the instrument measures what it is supposed to measure.

- **Content validity**
  Refers to an instrument's comprehensiveness, or how adequate the instrument reflects its purpose.

- **Face validity**
  Inferred from a panel of experts who evaluate the relevance of the content.

- **Criterion validity**
  Correlation with a "gold standard" measure of the same theme.

- **Predictive validity**
  Ability to predict a future state of affairs.

Methodology

- **Concurrent validity**
  Ability to accurately predict the current status of a situation or an individual compared to existing criterion (eg, another test).

- **Reliability**
  Ability of the instrument to measure something the same way twice.

- **Internal consistency**
  How consistent are the questions in measuring the same outcome?

- **Reproducibility**

- **Test-retest**
  How close are the results of an instrument given to the same patient on two different occasions?

- **Responsiveness**
  Ability of the instrument to change as the status of the patient changes.

- **Inter-observer**
  How closely does observer #1 agree with observer #2 using the same instrument on the same patient?

3 Clinical utility

- Patient friendliness
- Clinician friendliness

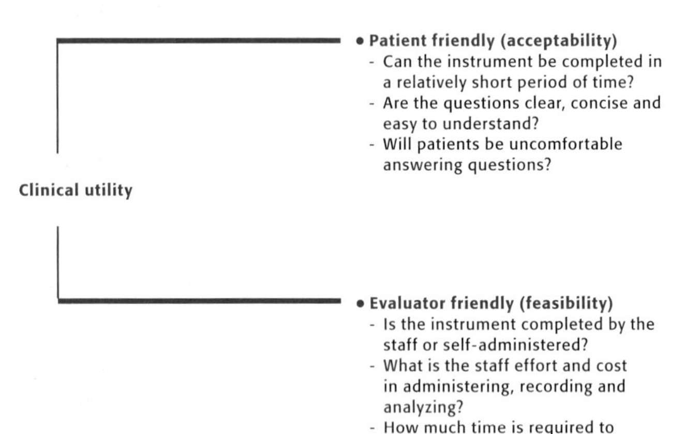

4 Scoring

After completion of our searching and summarizing, each instrument was then evaluated based on a 10 point scale and converted to the easy-to-use graphical representations contained herein. References are also clearly identified for the reader, should one be compelled to find the original work.

II Acknowledgements

The "AO Handbook of Musculoskeletal Outcomes Measures and Instruments" represents the dedication and hard work of several colleagues that must not go without acknowledgement.

To Joseph R Dettori, PhD, for his significant contribution to the development of the evaluation and scoring criteria of each instrument and chapter editing.

To Eric Strauss, MD, whose hard work as a medical student, in collecting the first round of outcomes instruments, made this book possible.

To Nate Dettori, BS, whose hard work in helping to search the literature and summarize content aided in the development and completion of this handbook.

To my co-authors Beate Hanson, MD, and Daniel Norvell, PhD, whose magnificent and tireless efforts helped to see this project through from the beginning.

To Urs Rüetschi, publisher extraordinaire for his ongoing confidence and attention to detail in making this handbook a reality.

To David Helfet, MD, teacher, mentor, and friend whose vigilant dedication to elevating the academic bar for orthopaedic surgeons was the inspiration for this project.

To the AO Foundation for generously supporting and funding this important project.

Michael Suk
December 2004

III Editors

Michael Suk, MD, JD, MPH
Assistant Professor
University of Florida
Director, Orthopaedic Trauma Service
Shands Jacksonville
655 West 8th Street
ACC Building, 2nd Floor/Ortho
US-Jacksonville, FL 32209

Beate P Hanson, MD, MPH
Assistant Professor
Director AO Clinical Investigation
and Documentation (AOCID)
Clavadelerstrase
CH-7270 Davos Platz

Daniel C Norvell, PhD
Clinical Epidemiologist
614 1st Street
US-Steilacoom, WA 98388

David L Helfet, MD, MBCHB
Profesor of Orthopaedic Surgery
Cornell University Medical College
535 East 70th Street
US-New York, NY 10021

1 Introduction

1 Current challenges

Words describing orthopedic outcomes are a natural part of our daily dialogue. Results described as "good" or "excellent" can be heard in physicians' offices, and rehabilitation clinics. These same descriptive terms are also replete in the musculoskeletal literature. But determining the exact meaning of these words and their relationship to reproducible results can be difficult.

In an attempt to move away from the vernacular and toward the scientific, researchers and clinicians have developed a variety of "outcomes instruments" to collect relevant data and to provide an "objective" basis for outcomes results. Today, previously used terms such as "good" and "excellent" are often used to describe a spectrum of outcomes that might reflect a mix of objective ("clinician based") results and subjective ("patient reported") scores that can be confusing, if not altogether unclear to most people.

Outcomes instruments can play an important role in the development of new procedures, techniques and protocols. The musculoskeletal literature is filled with clinical justifications based on outcomes nomenclature that can be at best difficult to verify and at worst, misleading. For example, how many of us truly know the 36 data points involved with an SF-36 instrument to feel truly comfortable with the determination of a "good" outcome? Further, without that requisite knowledge, how can we adequately assess one instrument over another? How often have you wished that you could quickly decipher an outcomes score without having to spend time looking up the original study?

2 The handbook

The "AO Handbook of Musculoskeletal Outcomes Measures and Instruments" is designed to provide the reader with a user-friendly and comprehensive summary of the major musculoskeletal outcomes instruments in use today.

The purpose is three-fold:

- To facilitate the use of outcomes instruments in daily clinical practice.
- To ease critical assessment of academic journal articles.
- To foster the development of new and improved outcomes instruments via standardized criteria.

3 The audience

The "AO Handbook of Musculoskeletal Outcomes Measures and Instruments" is intended for the use of any person involved in the treatment of musculoskeletal problems: orthopedic surgeons, physiatrists, rheumatologists, physical therapists, occupational therapists, family physicians, nurses, etc. Its detailed layout and color-coded indices are structured in a way to facilitate its use in everyday practice and research, while encouraging the use of a common terminology pertinent to all specialties.

It is our hope that by using this book, we can help to usher in a new era of clinical assessment, that is based on the appropriate marriage of science and epidemiology.

2 Why appropriate selection is important

1 Introduction

Taking into account the results of an appropriate outcomes instrument is a critical step in recommending a course of treatment for musculoskeletal care. This however, can be a challenging task. In the balance, one treatment protocol or intervention may be deemed better than another based on a specific desired endpoint (eg, range of motion), but not as good based on another endpoint (eg, pain relief.)

A well-designed study that clearly delineates superiority of one treatment over another may provide insufficient evidence or even be harmful if it fails to measure "important" outcomes.

Some of the best studies leave us with more questions because the authors failed to put thought into their outcome selection. For example, while one treatment method may lead to fewer short-term complications when compared to another, the same method may also result in decreased function or an inferior quality-of-life. Were these outcomes measured? What is critical to any clinical or research setting with respect to measuring treatment effectiveness, is identifying and measuring "important" outcomes. That which is deemed "important" may lie in the eye of the beholder; however, much thought should go into its definition. To understand the importance of appropriate outcomes selection, we must first understand the basic meaning of Outcomes Research.

2 Outcomes research

The purpose of this chapter is not to discuss the depth and breadth of Outcomes Research. That is beyond the scope of this Handbook; however, a basic understanding of its meaning and significance sets the stage for the selection of "important" outcomes measures and instruments. The need to know the actual value of health interventions in health care has led to the re-emergence of Outcomes

Research. It is important that we first consider the basic meaning of Outcomes Research before summarizing and evaluating the measures and instruments used. The following table is a sample of various definitions that exist for Outcomes Research:

The study of the end result of health services that take patient's experiences, preferences, and values into account [1].
"Outcomes Research is a wide spectrum of research activities that include assessment of treatment, measurement of treatment, and when that data is gathered, management of the treatment." [2]
The scientific study of the outcomes of disease therapies used for a particular disease, condition, or illness [3, 4].
Outcome research covers what the patient thinks of the results of the medical care he or she has been given; traditional research covers the standard evaluation of range of motion, strength, radiographs, etc. Outcomes research is in no way meant to replace the usual methods of research in the evaluation of treatment for musculoskeletal disease; it is meant to add another dimension for evaluation. [2]
The discipline that describes, interprets, the impact of various influences, especially interventions, on final endpoints (from survival to satisfaction with care) that matter to decision makers (from patients to society at large) [5].
A discipline dealing with research methods and efforts to measure what actually works (effectiveness) in health care using various complementary outcome measures, ranging from traditional clinical measures (symptom control, bony alignment, range of motion, disease progression or survival) to health-related quality of life and cost effectiveness measures [6, 7].

3 Outcomes, outcomes, and more outcomes

When a surgeon scrubs in to perform an orthopedic surgery, he or she is faced with the critical decision of which device or intervention strategy to use that best suits the patient's needs. For example, for proximal humerus fractures, there are nearly ten different implants available that purportedly serve the same function. If uninformed about the utility of each, this would be like viewing several identical closed doors and wondering what lies behind them. If informed, each closed door would have a different appearance that would indicate the strengths and limitations of each treatment method, making the decision of which door to open much easier for the surgeon.

Selecting an outcomes instrument is even more challenging. There are more than one hundred outcomes instruments available for selection in the musculoskeletal literature. For the shoulder joint alone, there are nearly 30 instruments to choose from and the list is growing. Knowing what lies behind each of these doors is a hurdle that cannot be overcome if left to search the literature on your own. With the aid of this book, you should be armed with the knowledge you need to make the appropriate selection.

4 Selecting important outcomes

This book will not tell you which outcome instrument you need for your specific situation. In the end, you must make that decision based on several factors. Selecting an important outcome is based on two important steps:

- Determine whether you are selecting the outcome for clinical or research purposes.
- Determine your clinical or study purpose(s).
- Determine what instruments are available that may address that purpose.
- Determine the quality of these instruments.

Following these steps will allow you to narrow your decision down to a manageable number of potential "important" outcomes instruments.

Once a set of measures and instruments has been identified, then their specific content, population intended for, and overall quality can be compared. Subsequent chapters will address how to evaluate the overall quality of an instrument.

5 Conclusion

With the pressure to approve and recommend specific devices and interventions to the musculoskeletal clinical and research community, Musculoskeletal Outcomes Research has a unique opportunity to demonstrate its ability to validate the true clinical benefit of these modalities in appropriate patient populations using appropriate measures and instruments as endpoints. Although the musculoskeletal literature has documented its importance, Outcomes Research has yet to demonstrate its role in the clinical and research settings and provide a comprehensive review of the validity, reliability, and responsiveness of those measures and instruments available for its application. Our hope is that this handbook will be a significant contributor to this endeavor.

6 References

[1] Clancy CM, Eisenberg JM (1998) Outcomes research: measuring the end results of health care. Science; 282: 245–246.
[2] Simmons BP, Swiontkowski MF, Evans RW, et al (1999) Outcomes assessment in the information age: available instruments, data collection, and utilization of data. Instr Course Lec;. 48: 667-85, 1999.
[3] Piccirillo JF (1994) Outcomes research and otolaryngology. Otolaryngol Head Neck Surg; 111: 764–769.
[4] Piccirillo JF, Stewart MG, Gliklich RE et al Outcomes research primer. Otolaryngol Head Neck Surg; 117:380–387.
[5] The outcomes of Cancer Outcomes Research Focusing on the National Cancer Institute's Quality-of-Care initiative. (2002) Med Care; 40:3–10.
[6] Anderson C (1994) Measuring what works in health care. Science; 3:1080.
[7] Epstein RS, Sherwood LM (1996) From outcomes research to disease management: a guide for the perplexed. Ann Intern Med; 124:832–837.

3 What makes a quality outcomes instrument?

Many factors must be taken into consideration when selecting or evaluating a "quality outcomes instrument". An explanation of these factors, including content, methods, and clinical utility, is the main focus of this chapter and is presented in the clear, consistent and accurate manner characteristic of this book. The concepts discussed in this chapter are the foundation for the overall evaluation of each instrument presented in chapter 6.

In assessing the overall quality of an outcomes instrument, three major components should be considered: content, methodology, and clinical utility.

1 Content

Simply defined, content is what the instrument is trying to measure. Are the instrument's questions relevant to your population of patients? Does the interpretation of the instrument's score make sense to you? The content of the instrument can be divided into three main categories: *type, scale* and *interpretation*.

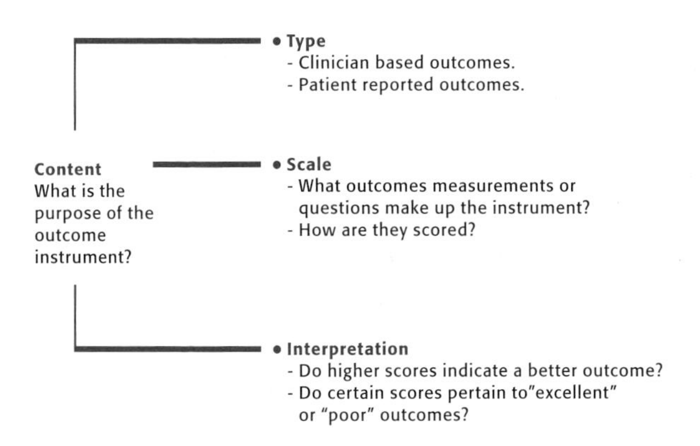

2 Methodology

The methodology of the instrument can be divided into three main categories: *validity, reliability,* and *responsiveness.*

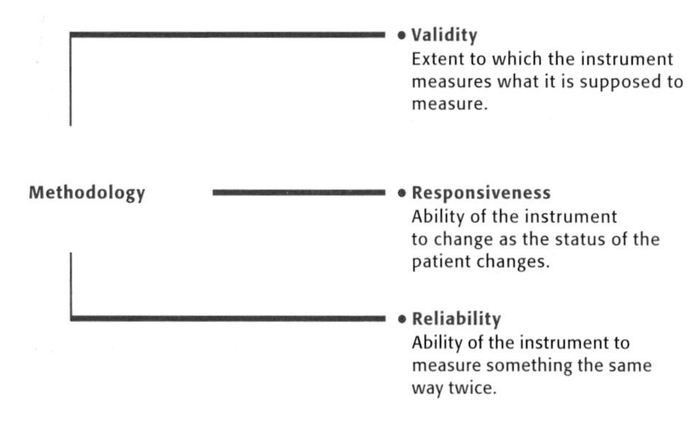

Validity is commonly defined as the extent to which an instrument measures what it is intended to measure. For example, in the sport of archery, validity would be represented by the accuracy of the shots—how close on average, do the shots come to the bull's eye of the target.

Reliability is concerned with the consistency of the instrument. In other words, it is the ability to measure something the same way twice. Using the archery example, reliability would be represented by how close successive shots are grouped together, wherever they hit the target.

Ideally, all shots land in the bull's eye of the target (valid and reliable). An archer who is consistently missing the bull's eye represented by a close grouping of shots somewhere on the periphery of the target is analogous to an instrument that is reliable but not valid.

Orthopedic residents learning trauma surgery must first learn to reduce a fracture successfully, and then learn to do this consistently. This is analogous to the validity and reliability of an outcomes instrument.

Responsiveness refers to the instrument's ability to change with the status of the patient. If a patient returns to work with some disability six months after surgery and progresses to full work with no disability after 12 months, an instrument that measures this patient's functional status should be sensitive enough to reflect this improvement.

What do we mean when we say an instrument is valid?

Because validity is not a fixed measure, an instrument should be considered valid for use in relation to a specific purpose or set of purposes [1] and in a specific patient population. For example, a valid measure of disability for patients with knee osteoarthritis following total knee arthroplasty cannot automatically be considered valid for use in patients with distal femoral fractures.
Furthermore, validity is not summed up by one concept but can be subdivided into the following concepts: *content, criterion,* and *construct validity*.

Validity can be further sub-divided into three main concepts.

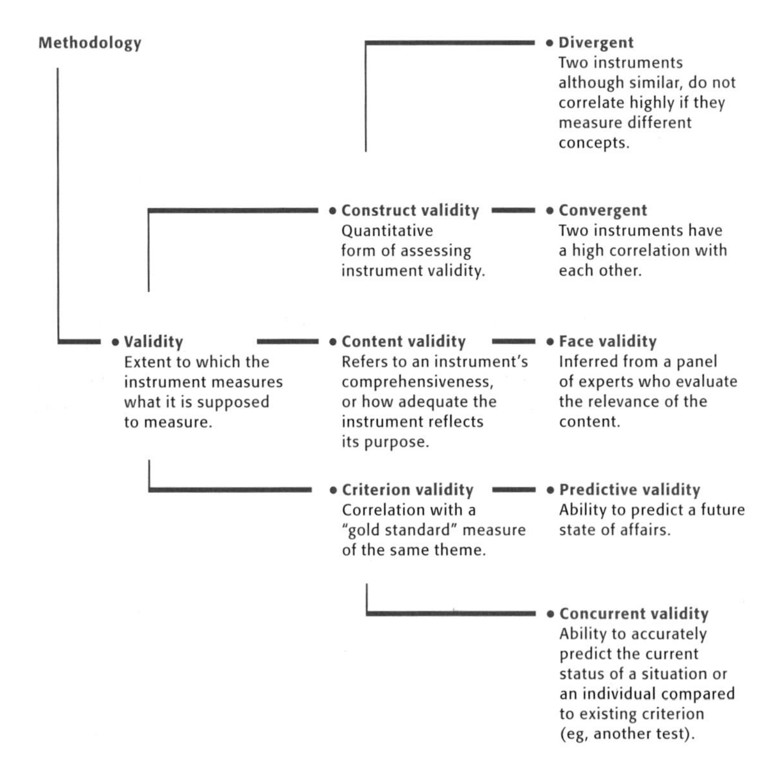

Content

Content validity refers to an instrument's comprehensiveness, or how adequately the questions included in the instrument (ie, its content) reflect its overall purpose. It has been described as a blend of common sense and technical psychometric properties [2]. For example, in a patient reported outcomes instrument designed for young patients with a knee injury, an instrument that asks about activities of daily living but ignores sporting activity may lack adequate content validity, leading to inaccurate conclusions.

Content validity is usually established by content experts: For a clinician based outcome that includes x-ray results, the physician or group of physicians are typically the experts for such clinical measures. On the other hand, for a patient reported outcomes that focus on health related quality-of-life, patients may be the experts.

Though it can be, content validity is rarely formally tested. Instead the *face validity* or clinical credibility of an instrument is commonly inferred from a panel of experts who evaluate the relevance of the content [1]. It is difficult, perhaps impossible, to prove formally that the items or questions chosen are representative of all relevant items [5].

Guyatt and colleagues differentiate content and face validity with the following statement: "Face validity examines whether an instrument appears to be measuring what it is intended to measure, and content validity examines the extent to which the domain of interest is comprehensively sampled by the items, or questions, in the instrument." [6]. Together they deal with whether the questions in an instrument address the intended subject matter and whether the full scope of the subject is adequately covered [1].

Face and content validity are best determined by examining the instrument. Another method of determining the content validity is to determine how the instrument was developed in the first place. How extensively did individuals with relevant clinical and methodology expertise participate in generating the content [7]? Perhaps even more important, to what extent did patients with experience of the health problem participate in creating and substantiating the content of an instrument [8]?

Criterion

Criterion validity considers whether an instrument correlates highly with a "gold standard" measure of the same theme* [1].
Criterion validity can be further sub-divided into concurrent and predictive validity.

Concurrent validity refers to an instrument's ability to accurately predict the current status of an individual. The instrument is compared to some already existing criterion (eg, another test). Criterion validity is the most concrete type of validity, and the type most often considered in traditional medical research [2]. Furthermore, if there is an external criterion against which to validate an instrument, it should be used. For example, a newly developed hip score for traumatic proximal femur fractures in younger adults may be compared to the nonarthritic hip score [3].

Predictive validity refers to an instrument's ability to predict a future status of an individual. For example, a specific cutoff from the injury severity score may be found to correlate highly with mortality within 30 days of the initial trauma.

* For measures of pain, quality of life, and depression, criterion validity is harder to demonstrate; validity testing is more challenging because there is rarely if ever a perfect "gold standard" against which to test the validity of a new outcomes instrument. However, there are a number of different and more indirect approaches recommended to judge instruments' validity [4]. Fitzpatrick and colleagues believe that "face, content, and construct validity are by far the most relevant issues for the use of patient reported outcomes measures in trials." [1].

Construct

Construct validity is a more quantitative form of assessing the validity of an instrument. A construct is an item or concept such as pain or disability. Individuals suffering more pain would be expected to take more pain medications. Individuals with more severe disability would be expected to have a greater limitation in range of motion or muscle strength. Construct validity is evaluated by quantitatively comparing the relationship of a construct like pain with another variable like pain medication use. For example, if you were to examine the validity of the scales of the Disabilities of the Shoulder Arm and Hand questionnaire (DASH) in patients with a distal radius fracture you would expect that the DASH physical function score should correlate most with the physical function scores of the SF-36, which is a general measure of physical, social, and emotional health. Conversely, measures of physical function would be expected to correlate less with measures of physical mood within the SF-36.

This highlights the two aspects of construct validity:

- convergent validity is represented when two instruments that measure similar concepts correlate highly with each other.
- divergent validity is represented when two instruments, although similar, do not correlate highly if they measure different concepts.

The important thing to recognize is that convergent and divergent validity work together. If you can demonstrate that there is evidence for both convergent and divergent validity, then there is evidence for construct validity. But, neither one alone is sufficient for establishing construct validity.

Demonstration of convergent and divergent validity requires the formulation of hypothesized relationships between the measure of interest and other measures of the same or distinctly different constructs. Once the hypothesized relationships have been established, then the measures of interest can be compared concurrently [9]. For example, to provide convergent and divergent evidence for validity for the International Knee Documentation Committee (IKDC) Subjective Knee Form, Irrgang and colleagues administered it concurrently with the SF-36 [9]. Because the IKDC Subjective Knee Form is a measure of physical function, they hypothesized that it would more strongly correlate with concurrent measures of physical function than to concurrent measures of mental function within the Short Form-36.

What do we mean when we say an instrument is reliable?

Reliability assesses the error in an instrument. In the archery analogy, reliability was symbolized by the shot grouping. Others have referred to this as "consistency," since reliability may be confused with "trustworthy" which would not be appropriate if an instrument repeatedly yields the wrong results [10].

Reliability is a very important property of any outcomes instrument when measuring the influence of an intervention. If an outcome is not reliable, changes observed in patients may not necessarily be attributed to the intervention, but rather, a problem inherent to the measuring instrument.

Like validity, reliability is not a fixed property, but is dependent upon the context of the population studied [11]. Reliability is best represented by *reproducibility* and *internal consistency*:

Reproducibility

There are two forms of reproducibility: inter-observer and test-retest.

Inter-observer reproducibility. Whenever you use humans as a part of your measurement procedure, you have to worry about whether the results you get are repeatable. People are notorious for their inconsistency. How closely observer #1 agrees with observer #2 using the same instrument and the same patient is the essence of inter-observer reproducibility.

This form of reproducibility is applicable to outcomes that are determined by a clinician (discussion on clinician based outcomes in chapter 4).

Test-retest reproducibility. Also known as intra-observer reproducibility. We estimate test-retest reproducibility when we administer the same instrument to the same patient on two different occasions. This approach assumes that there is no substantial change in the construct being measured between the two occasions. The amount of time allowed between measures is critical.

We know that if we measure the same thing twice that the correlation between the two observations will depend in part by how much time elapses between the two measurement occasions. The shorter the time gap, the higher the correlation; the longer the time gap, the lower the correlation.

Internal consistency

Internal consistency is a measure of how homogenous or consistent the questions in the scale are and to what extent they are measuring the same thing.

Most instruments employ several questions or items to assess a single construct or dimension (eg, pain, disability). This is because several related observations typically produce a more reliable estimate than one [1]. For this to hold true, the questions all need to be similar, measuring aspects of a single attribute [11].

The end result is that individual questions should correlate highly with each other and with the total score of items in the same scale. For example, a researcher designs a questionnaire to find out about how a young patient is performing in their job after returning to work following a motor vehicle accident that led to a severe tibial fracture. If similar questions pertaining to activities requiring the strength and repetitive use of the lower extremities score vastly different (some high some low), thereby rendering the internal consistency low, you would have to question the reliability of the instrument. On the other hand, if a patient consistently scores low in work-related activity questions pertaining to lower extremity function, the instrument is probably reliable with respect to that construct.

Internal consistency helps in addressing the inherent limitations of reproducibility. Often you cannot administer an instrument to your patients twice under the same circumstances. It's possible a patient could respond differently either because something has happened in their environment or self that might alter their response between evaluations, or they may remember answers they gave from the prior evaluation.

Reliability can be further sub-divided into two main concepts.

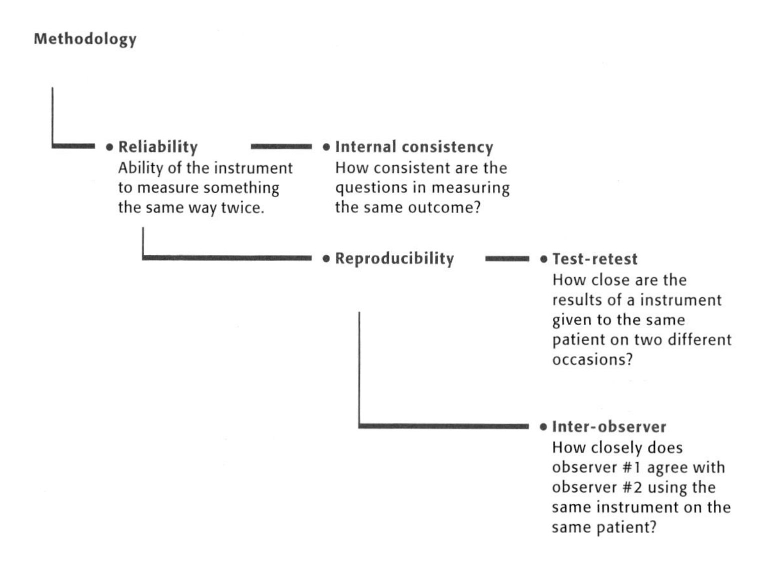

What do we mean when we say an instrument is responsive?

Responsiveness, also known as "sensitivity to change," is a measure of how well an instrument can detect changes as a result of an intervention [2]. It is possible for an instrument to be both valid and reliable but not responsive. This is problematic when applying an instrument to evaluate a patient's progress or the effects of a particular treatment.

A valid and reliable instrument that does not reflect changes as the patient gets worse or improves is of little clinical or research value.

The methodology of an instrument is defined by its validity, reliability, and responsiveness.

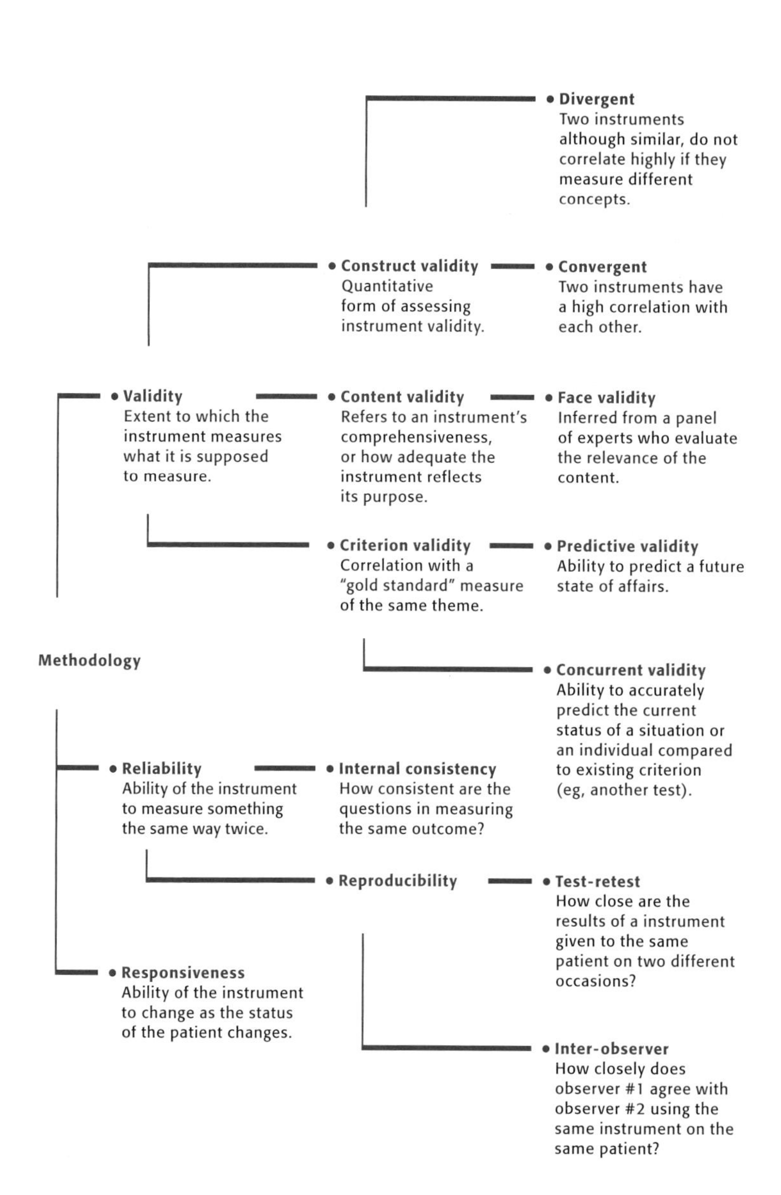
Methodology
• Validity
Extent to which the instrument measures what it is supposed to measure.
• Construct validity
Quantitative form of assessing instrument validity.
• Divergent
Two instruments although similar, do not correlate highly if they measure different concepts.
• Convergent
Two instruments have a high correlation with each other.
• Content validity
Refers to an instrument's comprehensiveness, or how adequate the instrument reflects its purpose.
• Face validity
Inferred from a panel of experts who evaluate the relevance of the content.
• Criterion validity
Correlation with a "gold standard" measure of the same theme.
• Predictive validity
Ability to predict a future state of affairs.
• Concurrent validity
Ability to accurately predict the current status of a situation or an individual compared to existing criterion (eg, another test).
• Reliability
Ability of the instrument to measure something the same way twice.
• Internal consistency
How consistent are the questions in measuring the same outcome?
• Reproducibility
• Test-retest
How close are the results of a instrument given to the same patient on two different occasions?
• Inter-observer
How closely does observer #1 agree with observer #2 using the same instrument on the same patient?
• Responsiveness
Ability of the instrument to change as the status of the patient changes.

3 Clinical utility

While an instrument may contain the appropriate content and demonstrate adequate methodology, it may be hard for the patient to complete or difficult for a clinician or researcher to administer or analyze. Therefore, we have included an additional subjective component to what makes a "quality outcomes measure" by including: *patient friendliness* and *clinician friendliness*.

What makes an instrument patient friendly?

It is essential that an instrument be acceptable to the patient to minimize patient burden [1]. There are two important reasons for this: to minimize any additional stress in patients already dealing with health problems and to ensure a high response rate to the questions in the instrument to make the data collected more easy to interpret, more generalizeable, and less prone to non-response bias.

Patient friendliness, also called acceptability, has been evaluated far less frequently than validity and reliability and there are no established standards for what constitutes this concept; nonetheless, it is certainly one that should be considered when selecting an appropriate outcomes instrument. We recommend you consider the following questions when determining patient friendliness. These questions are based on Selby and Robertson's definition [12]:

- Can the instrument be completed in a relatively short amount of time?
- Are the questions clear, concise, and easy to understand?
- Will patients be uncomfortable answering the questions?

Like the assessment of content validity, you may appropriately argue that patient friendliness should be evaluated by patients.

Sprangers and colleagues [13] argue that the patients' opinions should be assessed during the development phase of the instrument, prior to more formal tests of validity and reliability.

Ideally, when selecting an instrument, users should see evidence of this concept being evaluated during the design phase; however, this is rarely observed in musculoskeletal outcomes instruments.

What makes an instrument clinician friendly?

In addition to patient burden, it is important to consider the impact of administering an instrument on your staff and researchers who collect and process the information [14–16]. Also known as feasibility, we recommend you consider the following questions when determining clinician friendliness:

- Is this instrument completed by the staff or self administered?
- What is the staff effort and cost in administering, recording, and analyzing?
- How much time is required to train the staff in administering the instrument?

Read and colleagues [17] compared the training times required for the administration and management of three health status instruments and found that they varied from 1 to 2 hours for the easiest to 1 to 2 weeks for the most complex instrument.

It has been thought in the past that more complex scoring systems reduce the clinician friendliness compared to simple systems; however, with computer programs capable of processing large amounts of data in a short amount of time, this issue is less likely to play a major role on staff burden.

Bernard and colleagues summed this up nicely by arguing that staff attitudes and the acceptance of "quality" patient reported outcomes measures should make a significant difference in the ultimate acceptance by patients [18].

The clinical utility of an instrument can be divided into patient and clinician friendliness.

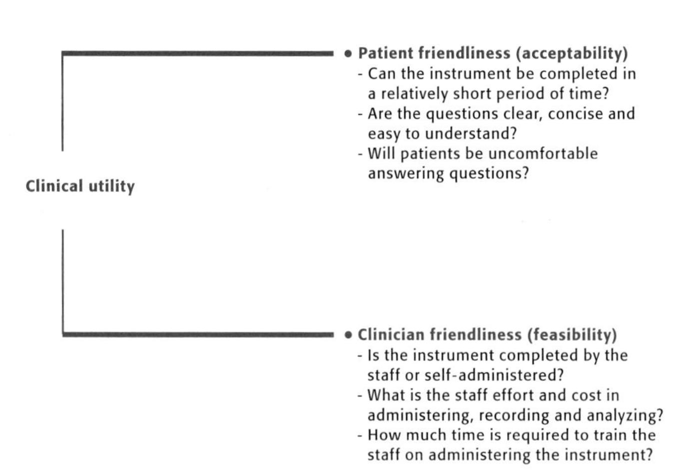

What type of instrument is important when considering clinical utility?

Since patient and clinician friendliness are intricately related, it behooves you to select an instrument that minimizes the burden for both groups. Although not the scope of this chapter, clinician based outcomes can put a much greater burden on clinical and research staff. In addition, there are good reasons to include patients in the evaluation of their outcomes (see chapters 4 and 5).

Hence, an instrument that involves little to no clinician effort to perform that maximizes the patient's assessment of their condition, without an undo burden on the patient, would arguably be the best instrument from a clinical utility and methodological standpoint. That said, we encourage the use of patient reported outcomes for both clinical and research purposes and this will be discussed in greater detail in subsequent chapters.

4 Assessing the overall quality of the instrument

Whether reading an article and evaluating its findings or selecting your own instrument to administer clinically or for research purposes, you must consider the many issues discussed in this chapter. It becomes a particular challenge as the number of potential instruments increases.

This book presents more than 150 possible outcomes instruments for the musculoskeletal extremities alone. How do you pick the right one?

In the end, it depends on the purpose of its use and the population for which it is intended. You need to first consider the content of the instrument. Does the scale address the appropriate questions for your population? Was anything left out? Is the interpretation of the overall score satisfying to you? Has the instrument been validated in a population in which you are interested? If so, how did it perform? Is it reliable and does it have the ability to demonstrate important clinical change after an intervention has been introduced? Will your patients and your staff find the instrument acceptable and feasible?

All these questions must be considered when comparing one instrument to another. It is not uncommon for one instrument to be better in certain situations but not as good in others. The relative merit of each instrument is addressed in this book by the application of an overall score based on the concepts addressed in this chapter.

The purpose of this book is to provide you the tools to help you make that final decision whether you are selecting an instrument or evaluating the results of a paper that uses one.

5 References

[1] Fitzpatrick R, Davey C, Buxton MJ, et al (1998) Evaluating patient-based outcome measures for use in clinical trials. Health Technol Assess; 2:1–74.
[2] Wassertheil-Smoller (1995) Mostly about quality of life. In: Biostatistics and Epidemiology, 2nd ed. New York: Springer-Verlag, pp. 147–155.
[3] Christensen CP, Althausen PL, Mittleman MA, et al (2003) The nonarthritic hip score: reliable and validated. Clin Orthop; 75–83.
[4] Partrick DL P. E (1993) Health Status and Health Policy. Oxford: Oxford University Press.
[5] Seiler LH (1973) The 22-item scale used in field studies of mental illness: a question of method, a question of substance, and a question of theory. J Health Soc Behav; 14: 252–64.
[6] Guyatt GH, Feeny DH, Patrick DL (1993) Measuring health-related quality of life. Ann Intern Med;118: 622–629.
[7] Guyatt GH, Cook DJ (1994) Health status, quality of life, and the individual. Jama; 272: 630–631.
[8] Lomas J, Pickard L, Mohide A (1987) Patient versus clinician item generation for quality-of-life measures. The case of language-disabled adults. Med Care; 25:764–769.
[9] Irrgang JJ, Anderson AF (2002) Development and validation of health-related quality of life measures for the knee. Clin Orthop; 402:95–109.
[10] Feinstein AR (1987) Clinimetrics. New Haven, Connecticut. Yale University Press.
[11] Streiner DL, Norman GR (1995) Health measurement scales: a practical guide to their development and use. 2nd ed. Oxford: Oxford University Press.
[12] Selby P, Robertson B (1987) Measurement of quality of life in patients with cancer. Cancer Surv; 6:521–543.
[13] Sprangers MA, Aaronson NK (1992) The role of health care providers and significant others in evaluating the quality of life of patients with chronic disease: a review. J Clin Epidemiol; 45:743–760.
[14] Aaronson NK (1992) Assessing the quality of life of patients in cancer clinical trials: Common problems and common sense solutions. Eur J Cancer; 1304.
[15] Lansky D, Butler JB, Waller FT (1992) Using health status measures in the hospital setting: from acute care to ‚outcomes management'. Med Care; 30:MS57–73.
[16] Erickson P, Taeuber RC, Scott J. (1995) Operational aspects of Quality-of-Life Assessment. Choosing the right instrument. Pharmacoeconomics; 7:39–48.
[17] Read JL, Quinn RJ, Hoefer MA (1987) Measuring overall health: an evaluation of three important approaches. J Chronic Dis; 40:7S–26S.
[18] Bernhard J, Gusset H, Hurny C (1995) Quality-of-life assessment in cancer clinical trials: an intervention by itself? Support Care Cancer; 3:66–71.

4 Clinician based outcomes measures

In evaluating an intervention or particular treatment protocol, students, physicians and researchers involved in musculoskeletal care have traditionally utilized several clinical parameters. Specifically, did the intervention or treatment protocol result in:

- An increased longevity?
- The prevention of deformity?
- Improved pain relief?
- The restoration or improvement of musculoskeletal function?
- The prevention of future functional decline?

Typically, outcomes that can be simply determined, such as increased longevity and deformity prevention are among the easiest to evaluate. Often, these outcomes do not require a written instrument to derive a conclusion. For example, a comparison of survival rates between elderly patients who sustain a hip fracture and undergo a particular intervention versus those who do not can be directly assessed and quantified.

On the other hand, evaluations of pain relief, functional improvement and the prevention of future functional decline is often more difficult to assess. These outcomes are frequently of great concern to the patient. As a result, clinicians have attempted to develop instruments that provide a measure of these outcomes by inference from either "clinician based" or "patient reported" outcomes instruments.

1 What are clinician based outcomes measures?

Clinician based outcomes (CBO) measures refer to an array of tests and measures that assess the result of healthcare interventions from the perspective of the clinician.

They are often physiologic and may include muscle strength, joint range of motion, gait abnormalities, bony alignment, edema, wound repair, response to provocative maneuvers, and clinician based inventories of physical/psychological/social function. They stand in contradistinction to patient reported outcomes (PRO) measures; those outcomes measures that reflect the patient's perception of their symptoms, functional ability, and quality-of-life.

2 Objectivity of clinician based outcomes measures

Previously, many CBO measures were considered "objective". After all, in most cases, the clinician was documenting the patient's progress directly, measuring motion, strength or other parameters that were deemed important. Outcome objectivity however, is not determined by whether a clinician measures a parameter directly, but rather, objectivity is dependent on the reliability or reproducibility of a finding, among patients and clinicians alike [1,2].

There remains substantial variability in many CBOs. For example, interobserver agreement in determining motion of the spine [3,4] or extremities [5–8] is often poor. Muscle strength can be difficult to reproduce, particularly manually [9], but also in some cases when a dynamometer is used [10–12]. Variability for simple imaging tests has also been documented [13,14].

Clinician based outcomes:

Clinician based outcomes are often physiologic and can be measured directly by the clinician.

Examples of clinician-based or physiologic outcomes include muscle strength, joint range of motion, gait abnormalities, limb length, and bony alignment.

These physiologic measures, often considered "hard" or "objective", frequently serve to infer functional ability.

Patient reported outcomes:

Patient reported outcomes are concerned with the patient's perception of their symptoms, functional ability, and quality-of-life.

They have been considered "soft" or "subjective", and there has been some reluctance in the past to place a high value on these determinations.

It is now generally agreed that a patient's symptoms, functional ability, and quality-of-life are important outcomes that also require direct assessment.

3 Clinician based outcomes measures and patient function

Historically, CBOs have enjoyed widespread use because of the fundamental assumption that physiologic outcomes and patient well-being are highly correlated. We now recognize however that this is not always true [15–18]. For example, it has been shown that only a weak association exists between radiographic severity of knee osteoarthritis and patient quality-of-life.*

Simple designations such as "excellent, good, fair, or poor" are commonly used to quantify outcomes, particularly in the musculoskeletal specialties. Assessments using these scales often presuppose a high correlation between *clinician based* physiologic outcomes with *patient reported* symptoms and functional status. For example, the Hospital for Special Surgery knee scale (HSS knee scale) combines pain, function, range of motion, strength, deformity and instability into a single score and classifies patients

* This was illustrated in a study where neither the measurement of mean joint space width (MJSW) nor the narrowest joint space point (NJSP) significantly correlated with pain, stiffness or function derived from a patient-reported outcome measure, the Western Ontario and McMaster Universities OA Index (WOMAC) [19]. In another example, 18 nonrheumatoid patients who underwent limited wrist fusion had wrist scores based on range of motion and grip strength that did not correlate highly with patient satisfaction or self-assessment of wrist performance [20].

into one of four categories mentioned above. In a direct comparison between the HSS knee scale and the Cincinnati knee rating system, Sgaglione et al [21] found that each would rate the same patients differently. The proportion of subjects rated as excellent ranged from 23% (Cincinnati) to 76% (HSS knee scale).

The Thompson and Epstein score [22] for hip evaluation combines clinical and radiographic scores. Their clinical score identifies the following grades:

Excellent	No pain No limp Full hip motion
Good	No pain Slight limp At least 75% of normal hip motion
Fair	Pain, but not disabling Antalgic gait Moderate limitation of hip motion
Poor	Disabling pain Marked limitation of hip motion Adduction contracture Redislocation

This scale again classifies patients into four categories that only identify gross differences in function. Furthermore, the rating system combines symptoms, gait, motion and hip dislocation within a single rating, despite the fact that these outcomes may vary independently. For example, what is the grade if the patient has no pain but marked limitation of hip motion and does not dislocate?

In summary, CBOs are not necessarily more objective than PROs, nor are they necessarily related to a patient's relief of symptoms, functional ability, and quality-of-life. Older clinician based scales that combine clinical measures and patient symptoms can cause confusion, especially when simple designations are used to summarize the scale.

4 References

[1] Feinstein AR (1977) Clinical biostatistics. XLI. Hard science, soft data, and the challenges of choosing clinical variables in research. Clin Pharmacol Ther; 22:485–498.

[2] Deyo RA (1998) Using outcomes to improve quality of research and quality of care. J Am Board Fam Pract; 11:465–473.

[3] Nelson MA, Allen P, Clamp SE, et al (1979) Reliability and reproducibility of clinical findings in low-back pain. Spine; 4:97–101.

[4] Miller SA, Mayer T, Cox R, et al (1992) Reliability problems associated with the modified Schober technique for true lumbar flexion measurement. Spine; 17:345–348.

[5] Edwards TB, Bostick RD, Greene CC, et al (2002) Interobserver and intraobserver reliability of the measurement of shoulder internal rotation by vertebral level. J Shoulder Elbow Surg; 11:40–42.

[6] Hoving JL, Buchbinder R, Green S, et al (2002) How reliably do rheumatologists measure shoulder movement? Ann Rheum Dis; 61:612–616.

[7] Youdas JW, Bogard CL and Suman VJ (1993) Reliability of goniometric measurements and visual estimates of ankle joint active range of motion obtained in a clinical setting. Arch Phys Med Rehabil; 74:1113–1118.

[8] Bovens AM, van Baak MA, Vrencken JG, et al (1990) Variability and reliability of joint measurements. Am J Sports Med; 18:58–63.

[9] Hayes K, Walton JR, Szomor ZL, et al (2002) Reliability of 3 methods for assessing shoulder strength. J Shoulder Elbow Surg; 11:33–39.

[10] Moller M, Lind K, Styf J, et al (2003) The reliability of isokinetic testing of the ankle joint and a heel-raise test for endurance. Knee Surg Sports Traumatol Arthrosc; 22:22.

[11] Moreland J, Finch E, Stratford P, et al (1997) Interrater reliability of six tests of trunk muscle function and endurance. J Orthop Sports Phys Ther; 26:200–208.

[12] Agre JC, Magness JL, Hull SZ, et al (1087) Strength testing with a portable dynamometer: reliability for upper and lower extremities. Arch Phys Med Rehabil; 68:454–458.

[13] Koran LM (1975) The reliability of clinical methods, data and judgments (second of two parts). N Engl J Med; 293:695–701.

[14] Deyo RA, McNiesh LM and Cone RO (1985) 3rd: Observer variability in the interpretation of lumbar spine radiographs. Arthritis Rheum; 28:1066–1070.
[15] Torgerson WR and Dotter WE (1976) Comparative roentgenographic study of the asymptomatic and symptomatic lumbar spine. J Bone Joint Surg Am; 58:850–853.
[16] Witt I, Vestergaard A and Rosenklint A (1984) A comparative analysis of x-ray findings of the lumbar spine in patients with and without lumbar pain. Spine; 9:298–300.
[17] Wilson IB and Cleary PD (1995) Linking clinical variables with health-related quality of life. A conceptual model of patient outcomes. Jama; 273:59–65.
[18] Khan AM, McLoughlin E, Giannakas K, et al (2004) Hip osteoarthritis: where is the pain? Ann R Coll Surg Engl; 86:119–121.
[19] Bruyere O, Honore A, Rovati LC, et al (2002) Radiologic features poorly predict clinical outcomes in knee osteoarthritis. Scand J Rheumatol; 31:13–16.
[20] Tomaino MM, Miller RJ and Burton RI (1994) Outcome assessment following limited wrist fusion: objective wrist scoring versus patient satisfaction. Contemp Orthop; 28:403–410.
[21] Sgaglione NA, Del Pizzo W, Fox JM, et al (1995) Critical analysis of knee ligament rating systems. Am J Sports Med; 23:660–667.
[22] Thompson VP and Epstein HC (1951) Traumatic dislocation of the hip; a survey of two hundred and four cases covering a period of twenty-one years. J Bone Joint Surg Am.

5 The purpose of patient reported outcomes

1 What are patient reported outcomes?

For the purpose of this book, by patient reported outcomes (PRO) we mean questionnaires or instruments that patients complete by themselves or, when necessary, others on their behalf to obtain information in relation to functional ability, symptoms, health status, health-related quality of life, and results on specific treatment strategies. There is now a large array of such instruments available for musculoskeletal conditions, many of which are evaluated in chapter 6.

2 The emergence of patient reported outcomes

It is increasingly recognized that traditional clinician based outcomes measures (discussed in chapter 4) need to be complemented by measures that focus on the patient's concerns in order to evaluate interventions and identify whether one treatment is better than another [1].

Interest in PROs has been fueled by an increased importance of chronic conditions, where the objectives of treatment are to restore or improve function while preventing future functional decline [2]. The PROs typically measured in outcomes research are health-related quality of life, symptoms, and functional status [3].

There are no standards for each of those terms; however, outcomes researchers agree that quality of life is more important than the absence of a deformity or disease. It is multidimensional and should be from the patient's perspective [4,5].

3 Types of instruments

Patient reported outcomes are classified as either general (generic) or disease-specific measures of health-related quality of life. General measures are designed to be used across different diseases and across different demographic and cultural subgroups [6]. They are usually multidimensional and are designed to give a comprehensive and general overview of health-related quality of life.

The most well known general measure of health-related quality of life is the Short Form 36 health survey questionnaire [7]; typically known as the "SF-36". General measures of health-related quality of life permit comparisons across populations with different health conditions [8] and are more likely to detect unexpected effects of an intervention [6,8]. An important limitation is that they tend to be less responsive (concept discussed in chapter 3) than specific measures of health-related quality of life to changes in health status [9,10] and therefore less likely to detect the effects of a specific intervention.

Musculoskeletal disease-specific measures of health-related quality of life, on the other hand, focus on aspects of health that are specific to an injury (eg, fracture), disease (eg, osteoarthritis), anatomic area (eg, knee), or population of interest (eg, athletes). Several advantages are reported for disease-specific measures [11].

First, they were developed to have very relevant content when used with a specific disease or region of the body. This specificity has been shown to contribute to a more responsive measure [9,10]. Generally, they are more able to detect smaller or important changes that occur over time in the particular disease studied [6,12].

Second, this specificity has been shown to contribute to a more responsive measure [9,10]. A hip-specific instrument designed for patients with osteoarthritis should be particularly responsive to important changes in patients receiving total hip arthroplasty because it focuses only on the most relevant items.

Third, assuming the instrument has clear relevance to the patient's health problem [11], it might also be argued that greater patient acceptance leads to higher response and data collection rates.

An important limitation of musculoskeletal disease-specific measures is that it is generally not possible to administer them to patients who do not have the relevant disease or health condition.

This is a problem when investigators are interested in data from a general health sample of individuals to compare outcomes with a study sample. Furthermore, they do not allow for an easy comparison to be made between outcomes of different treatments for patients with different health conditions.

This is only a problem when the effectiveness of treatment regimes is necessary for purposes such as resource allocation [13]. Finally, it's also possible that the only available disease-specific instruments were developed in populations for purposes different than the disease or condition of interest. For example, several knee-specific PROs exist, most of which were developed in elderly patients with osteoarthritis or young patients with ligamentous sports injuries. No instruments exist that were developed for young patients with traumatic fractures of the distal femur or proximal tibia.

If resources allow, it is recommended that both a generic and disease-specific patient reported outcomes measure be administered to ensure an adequate assessment of a patient's entire health-related quality of life [14,15]. For example, in an assessment of construct validity among patients aged 67–99 years who had undergone knee replacement surgery, the WOMAC was found to discriminate better among individuals with knee problems, while the SF-36 discriminated better among individuals with varying levels of self reported general health status and comorbidities [16].

These results support inclusion of both a generic and a disease-specific PRO. However, one must consider the disadvantages of administering more than one instrument.

First, an additional instrument may increase the patient burden thereby reducing overall compliance.

Second, additional instruments increase the burden on the staff that is collecting and analyzing these data.

Furthermore, increasing the frequency of statistical analyses may give rise to statistically significant effects that arise by chance, although this can be remedied by stating hypotheses up front before conducting a study.

4 References

[1] Slevin ML, Plant H, Lynch D, et al (1988) Who should measure quality of life, the doctor or the patient? Br J Cancer; 57:109–112.

[2] Byrne M (1992) Cancer chemotherapy and quality of life. Bm; 304:1523–1524.

[3] 0Stewart MG, Neely JG, Hartman JM, et al (2002) Tutorials in clinical research: part V: outcomes research. Laryngoscope; 112:248–254.

[4] Gill TM, Feinstein AR (1994) A critical appraisal of the quality of quality-of-life measurements. Jama; 272:619–626.

[5] Cella DF, Bonomi AE (1995) Measuring quality of life: 1995 update. Oncology; 9:47–60.

[6] McSweeny AJ, Creer TL (1995)Health-related quality-of-life assessment in medical care. Dis Mon; 41:1–71.

[7] Ware JE Jr, Sherbourne CD (1992) The MOS 36-item short-form health survey (SF-36). I. Conceptual framework and item selection. Med Care; 30:473–483.

[8] Kessler RC, Mroczek DK (1995) Measuring the effects of medical interventions. Med Care; 33AS: 109–119.

[9] Guyatt GH, Feeny DH, Patrick DL (1993) Measuring health-related quality of life. Ann Intern Med; 118:622–629.

[10] Wright JG, Young NL (1997) A comparison of different indices of responsiveness. J Clin Epidemiol; 50:239–246.

[11] Fitzpatrick R, Davey C, Buxton MJ, et al (1998) Evaluating patient-based outcome measures for use in clinical trials. Health Technol Assess; 2:1–74.

[12] Patrick DL, Deyo RA (1989) Generic and disease-specific measures in assessing health status and quality of life. Med Care; 27:217–232.

[13] Cairns J (1996) Measuring health outcomes. Bmj; 313:6.
[14] Fletcher A, Gore S, Jones D, et al (1992) Quality of life measures in health care. II: Design, analysis, and interpretation. Bmj; 305:1145–1148.
[15] Guyatt G, Feeny D, Patrick D (1991) Issues in quality-of-life measurement in clinical trials. Control Clin Trials; 12:81S-90S.
[16] Hawker G, Melfi C, Paul J, at al (1995) Comparison of a generic (SF-36) and a disease specific (WOMAC) (Western Ontario and McMaster Universities Osteoarthritis Index) instrument in the measurement of outcomes after knee replacement surgery. J Rheumatol; 22:1193–1196.
[17] Till JE, Sutherland HJ, Meslin EM (1992) Is there a role for preference assessments in research on quality of life in oncology? Qual Life Res; 1:31–40.
[18] Roos E (2000) Rigorous statistical reliability, validity, and responsiveness testing of the Cincinnati Knee Rating System in 350 subjects with uninjured, injured, or anterior cruciate ligament-reconstructed knee. Am J Sports Med; 28:436–438.

6 Musculoskeletal outcomes measures and instruments

1 How the outcomes are displayed in this book

The purpose of this book is to provide the clinician or researcher with a user-friendly display of the most common disease-specific musculoskeletal outcomes, and a few common generic measures, all in one quick-reference location.

For simplicity, each instrument is displayed on two side-by-side pages containing:

- A summary of its content.
- A summary of any validity, reliability, or responsiveness evaluations with corresponding patient populations.
- A score for clinical utility based on our patient friendly and clinician friendly scoring criteria.
- An overall score.

The summary of the content is reflective of both the content of the instrument and the authors' description of the instrument. In cases where this information was not readily clear, every effort was made to contact the corresponding author of the instrument to clarify content related issues.

Where applicable, the section summary references the outcomes and populations against which the instrument was validated; otherwise, the term "not tested" is used. A "+" indicates the concept was judged favorably (eg, valid) and a "-" indicates that it was judged unfavorably (eg, not valid). A "+/-" indicates that one sub-component of the concept was favorable and another sub-component was unfavorable (eg, it demonstrated criterion validity but failed to demonstrate construct validity). This occurred rarely but nonetheless is reported when identified.

The clinical utility evaluation was performed by a team of individuals who reviewed and scored each instrument based on consensus criteria for patient friendliness and clinician friendliness.

With respect to whether the instrument was deemed patient friendly, the following questions were considered:

- Can the instrument be completed in a short amount of time?
- Are the questions clear, concise, and easy to understand?
- Will patients be uncomfortable answering the questions?

With respect to whether the instrument was deemed clinician friendly, the following questions were considered:

- Is this instrument completed by the staff or self-administered?
- What is the staff effort and cost in administering, recording, and analyzing?
- How much time is required to train the staff in administering the instrument?

Each instrument received a score between 0 to 10 points. Six possible points corresponded to the *methodological evaluation* and four possible points corresponded to the *clinical utility evaluation*. Each methodological concept received "no points", "0 points", or "1 point", which corresponded to whether the concept was found "not tested", "unfavorable" (eg, not valid) or "favorable" (eg, valid), respectively:

no points	"not tested"
0 point	"unfavorable"
1 points	"favorable"

Each clinical utility concept received "0 points", "1 point", or "2 points", which corresponded to whether the concept was found "limited", "moderate", or "strong", respectively:

no points	"limited"
0 point	"moderate"
1 points	"strong"

The *methodological evaluation, clinical utility,* and *overall score* sections were summarized by a "bubble score" depicting the number of points it received out of the total points possible for each corresponding section.

2 How to use the overall score

The overall score has its inherent limitations. It is not necessarily true that each concept evaluated should be equally weighted. However, since users will disagree on which principles are more important, we chose to use equal weighting for the methodological concepts as a reasonable alternative.

Since we felt that the clinical utility was very important in the overall merit of the instrument, the two concepts were given greater weight in an attempt to "even up" the two sections. In the end, the methodological evaluation contributes 60%, and the clinical utility evaluation contributes 40% to the overall score.

A higher score does not necessarily mean that the instrument is the best outcome instrument to use in all situations. Clinicians should consider their population of interest with respect to joint(s) involved, disease or injury incurred, and demographics.

These must be compared with the population in which the outcome instrument was created and tested. For example, if the population of interest is young and active, an instrument that was developed and tested in an elderly population that receives a score of 8 out of 10 may be less appropriate than one developed for a younger population that scores 6 out of 10.

Furthermore, clinicians should consider what the instrument was validated against. Though there are few "gold standards" in this area, some instruments are inherently stronger than others, so that should be taken into consideration.

Consequently, the score should not stand alone in the decision making process. The user should first understand for what and for whom the instrument was developed. The score can then be applied when trying to determine which one is most appropriate or superior in a given situation.

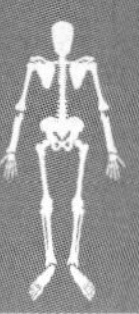

6.1 Generic instruments

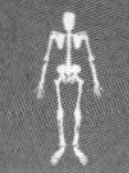

1. Musculoskeletal Function Assessment (MFA) (1996)

Source: Martin DP, Engelberg R, Agel J, Snapp D, Swiontkowski MF (1996) Development of a musculoskeletal extremity health status instrument: the Musculoskeletal Function Assessment instrument. J Orthop Res; 14:173–181.

Content

Type Generic patient reported outcome
Scale 10 categories (100 items):

Self-care (18 items)
Sleep and rest (6 items)
Hand and fine motor skills (7 items)
Mobility (20 items)
Housework (9 items)
Employment and work (4 items)
Leisure and recreational activities (4 items)
Family relationships (10 items)
Cognition and thinking (4 items)
Emotional adjustment, coping, and adaptation (18 items)

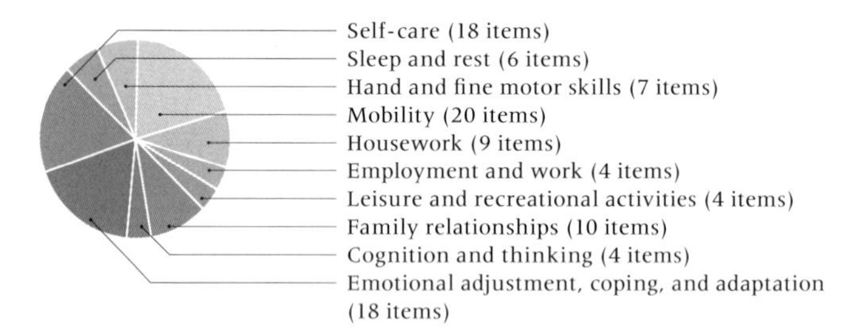

Patients assess their function by answering "yes" (1 point) or "no" (0 points) to each item of the questionnaire.

Interpretation

Raw category score = sum of all yes/no items within a category.
Raw MFA score = sum of all 100 yes/no items or sum of raw category scores.

Standardized category score = (raw category score/number of items in category) × 100

The MFA score = (raw MFA score/100) × 100

Note: the raw MFA score = the MFA score since the MFA has 100 items.

Minimum score: 0 points
Maximum score: 100 points

The higher the score, the lower the function.

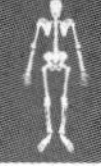

2. Nottingham Health Profile (NHP) (1981)

Source: Hunt SM, McKenna SP, McEwen J, Williams J, Papp E (1981): The Nottingham Health Profile: subjective health status and medical consultations.
Soc Sci Med [A]; 15:221–229.

Content

Type Generic patient reported outcome
Scale 6 subscales (38 items):

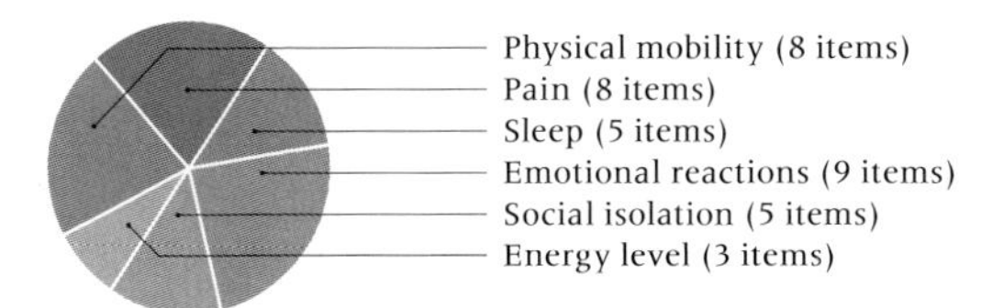

Each item is answered "yes" or "no".

Total score for each subscale is based on the percentage of items affirmed (ie, "yes") in each subscale.

Interpretation
Each subscale scored separately.

Overall score is the mean across all subscales.

Minimum score: 0 points
Maximum score: 100 points

The higher the score, the lower the function.

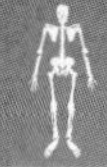

3. Short Form 36 health survey questionnaire (SF-36)* (1992)

Source SF-36: Ware JE Jr, Sherbourne CD (1992) The MOS 36-item short-form health survey (SF-36). I. Conceptual framework and item selection. Med Care; 30:473–483.
Source SF-12: Ware J Jr, Kosinski M, Keller SD (1996) A 12-Item Short-Form Health Survey: construction of scales and preliminary tests of reliability and validity. Med Care; 34:220–233.

Other versions available: SF-12, SF-8
Both shorter versions measure the same 8 subscales with fewer items.

Content

Type Generic patient reported outcome
Scale 8 subscales measuring physical and mental health (36 items):

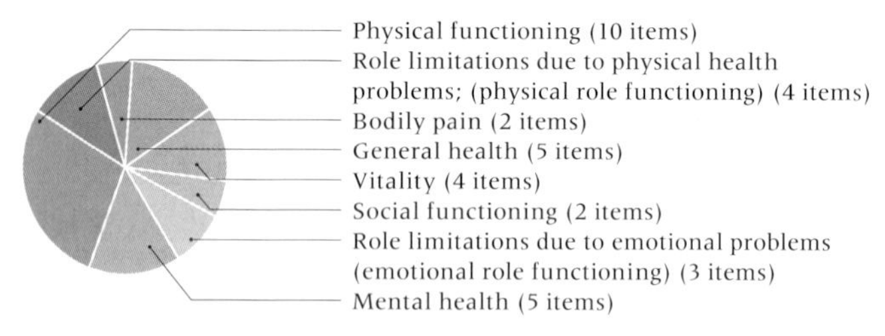

Reported health transition (1 item) is used to measure changes in health status. It is not included in any of the subscales and is administered as a supplemental question.

Interpretation

The questionnaire provides 8 subscale scores but not a total score.

For each subscale:
Minimum score: 0 points; maximum score: 100 points

The higher the score, the higher the function.

Norm-based scoring (NBS) can be used to score all 3 SF surveys. Through NBS, scale and summary scores are standardized to a mean of 50 and a standard deviation of 10 in the general US population, allowing scores to be compared within and across the different SF surveys.

** The SF-36 and SF-12 are available in original (SF-36 and SF-12) and updated (SF-36v2 and SF-12v2) versions, while the SF-8 is available in one version only. Versions 2.0 are very similar to versions 1.0; however, they offer a number of improvements, including increased range and precision for the role-functioning scales, improved item wording, and an easier-to-use format.*

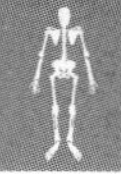

4. Short Musculoskeletal Function Assessment (SMFA) (1999)

Source: Swiontkowski MF, Engelberg R, Martin DP, Agel J (1999) Short musculoskeletal function assessment questionnaire: validity, reliability, and responsiveness.
J Bone Joint Surg Am; 81:1245–1260.

Content

Type Generic patient reported outcome
Scale Two indices (46 items):
"Dysfunction index" (34 items) and "bother index" (12 items).

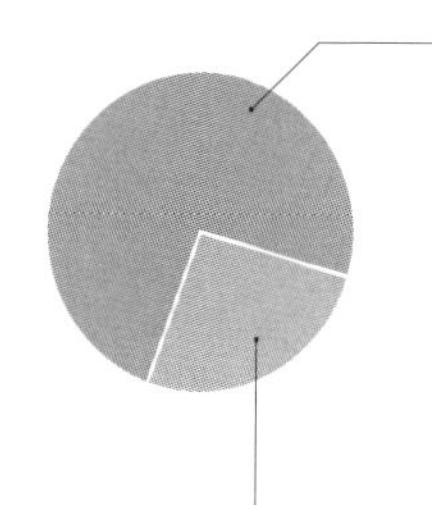

Dysfunction index (34 items):
- Amount of difficulty one has performing certain functions (25 items)
- How often one has difficulty when performing certain functions (9 items)

Functions are divided into the following 4 categories:
- Daily activities
- Emotional status
- Function of the arm and hand
- Mobility

Bother index (12 items):
Allows patients to assess how much they are bothered by problems in the following broad functional areas:
- Recreation and leisure
- Sleep and rest
- Work
- Family

Each item scored on 1 to 5-point Likert scale.

Interpretation

Item responses are summed then scores are normalized to a range of 0 to 100 points with the following formula:

([actual raw score - lowest possible raw score]/possible range of raw score) × 100

The higher the score, the lower the function.

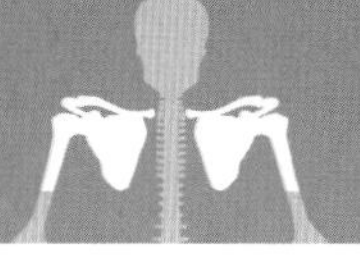

6.2 Shoulder

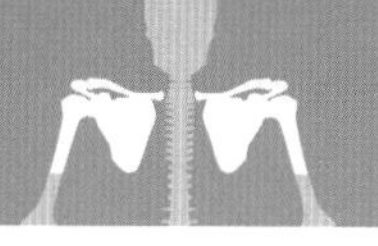

1. American Shoulder and Elbow Society Scoring system (ASES) (1994)

Richards RR, A. KN., Bigliani LU, Friedman RJ, Gartsman GM, Gristina AG, et al (1994) A standardized method for the assessment of shoulder function.
J Shoulder Elbow Surg; 3:347.

Content

Type Clinician based outcome
Scale 2 subscales (46 items):

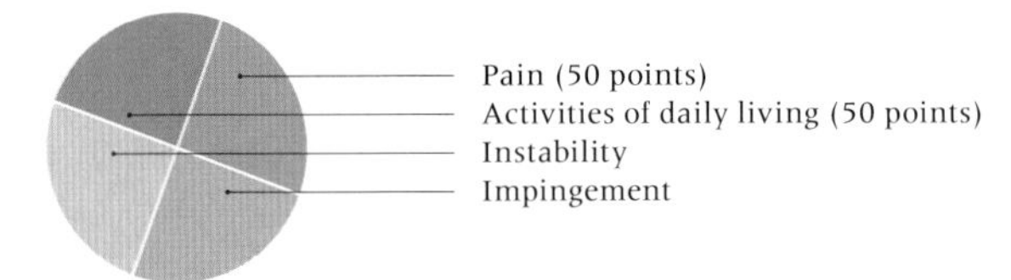

[(10 - pain score) × 5] + [(5/3) × ADL Score]= Shoulder Score Index (SSI)

Instability and impingement (clinical and patient-reported) do not contribute to the total score

Interpretation

Minimum score: 0 points
Maximum score: 100 points

The higher the score, the higher the function.

Validation

Outcomes validated against [1]

- SSRS
- SPADI
- SST
- Shoulder severity index
- SF-36

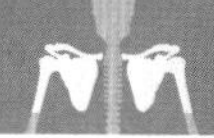

Validation (cont)

Outcomes validated against [2]
- Constant-Murley shoulder score
- VAS for satisfaction

Outcomes validated against [3]
- SANE
- Rowe shoulder score

Patient population tested in	Validity	Reliability	Responsiveness
Patients who underwent rotator cuff surgery or total shoulder arthroplasty (55 years; 59% male) [1]	not tested	not tested	+
Patients expected to be stable in their shoulder function (48 years; 45% male) [1]	not tested	+	not tested
Patients with combined tears of supraspinatus and infraspinatus (55.3 years; 70% male) [2]	+	not tested	not tested
Patients who underwent shoulder surgery for instability or significant AC separations (20 years; 90% male) [3]	+	not tested	+
Patients with shoulder dysfunction (49.2 years; 65% male) [4]	not tested	+	not tested
Subjects without a history of shoulder injury or surgery (42.8 years; 54% male) [5]	not tested	+	not tested

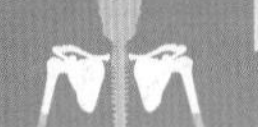

Validation (cont)

Validation studies:

[1] Beaton D., Richards RR (1998) Assessing the reliability and responsiveness of 5 shoulder questionnaires. J Shoulder Elbow Surg; 7:565–572.

[2] Skutek M, Fremerey RW, Zeichen J, et al (2000) Outcome analysis following open rotator cuff repair. Early effectiveness validated using four different shoulder assessment scales. Arch Orthop Trauma Surg; 120:432–436.

[3] Williams GN, Gangel TJ, Arciero RA, et al (1999) Comparison of the Single Assessment Numeric Evaluation method and two shoulder rating scales. Outcomes measures after shoulder surgery. Am J Sports Med; 27:214–221.

[4] Cook KF, Roddey TS, Olson SL, et al (2002) Reliability by surgical status of self-reported outcomes in patients who have shoulder pathologies. J Orthop Sports Phys Ther; 32:336–346.

[5] Sallay PI, Reed L (2003) The measurement of normative American Shoulder and Elbow Surgeons scores. J Shoulder Elbow Surg; 12:622–627.

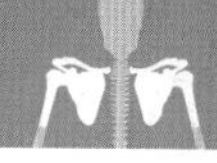

1. American Shoulder and Elbow Society Scoring system (ASES) (1994)

Methodological evaluation ●●●●●○ (5/6)

		no score	0 points	1 point	points
Validity	Content validity	not tested	not valid	**valid**	1
Validity	Construct validity	**not tested**	not valid	valid	-
Validity	Criterion validity	not tested	not valid	**valid**	1
Reliability	Internal consistency	not tested	not consistent	**consistent**	1
Reliability	Reproducibility	not tested	not reproducible	**reproducible**	1
	Responsiveness	not tested	not responsive	**responsive**	1
				Subtotal	**5**

Clinical utility ●●○○ (2/4)

	0 points	1 point	2 points	points
Patient friendliness	limited	moderate	**strong**	2
Clinician friendliness	**limited**	moderate	strong	0
			Subtotal	**2**

Total (out of 10) ●●●●●●●○○○ **7**

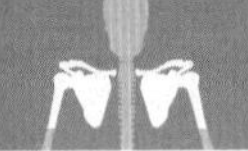

2. Athletic shoulder outcome scoring system (1993)

Source: Tibone JE, B. J (1993) Evaluation of treatment outcomes for the athlete's shoulder. In: The shoulder: a balance of mobility and stability.
Edited by F. F, Matsen FA, Hawkins RJ; Rosemont, IL: American Academy of Orthopedic Surgeons.

Content

Type Clinician based outcome
Scale 6 subscales:

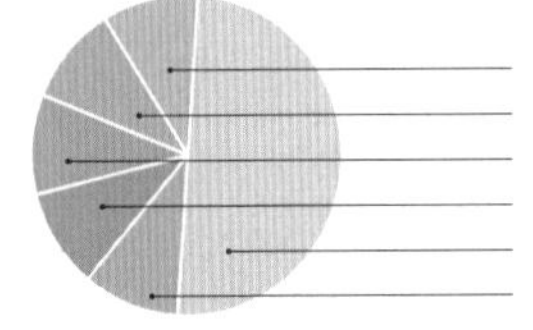

Pain (10 points)
Strength/endurance (10 points)
Stability (10 points)
Intensity (10 points)
Performance (50 points)
Range of motion (10 points)

Interpretation
Excellent: 90–100 points
Good: 70–89 points
Fair: 50–69 points
Poor: < 50 points

Validation

No validation studies were identified.

Patient population tested in	Validity	Reliability	Responsiveness
Not applicable			

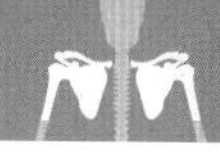

Methodological evaluation ○○○○○○ (0/6)

		no score	0 points	1 point	points
Validity	Content validity	not tested	not valid	valid	-
	Construct validity	not tested	not valid	valid	-
	Criterion validity	not tested	not valid	valid	-
Reliability	Internal consistency	not tested	not consistent	consistent	-
	Reproducibility	not tested	not reproducible	reproducible	-
	Responsiveness	not tested	not responsive	responsive	-
				Subtotal	-

Clinical utility ●●●○ (3/4)

	0 points	1 point	2 points	points
Patient friendliness	limited	moderate	strong	2
Clinician friendliness	limited	moderate	strong	1
			Subtotal	3

Total (out of 10) ●●●○○○○○○○ **3**

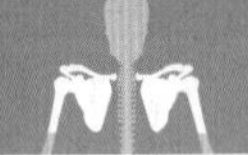

3. Constant-Murley functional assessment of the shoulder (1987)

Source: Constant CR, Murley AH (1987)
A clinical method of functional assessment of the shoulder.
Clin Orthop (214);160–164.

Content

Type Clinician based outcome
Scale 4 subscales (10 items):

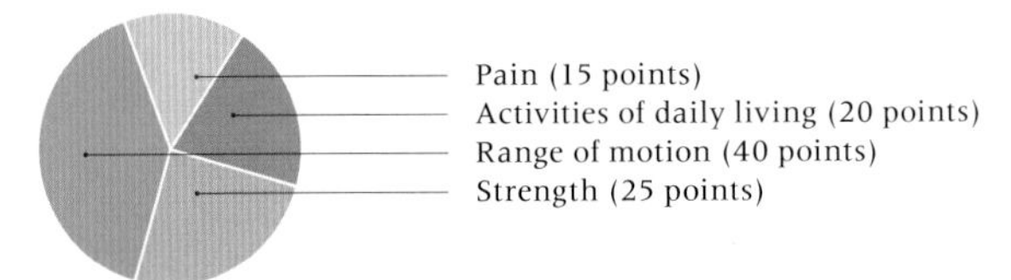

Modified score: strength assessed with sling over upper arm.
Abbreviated score: excludes strength assessment.

Interpretation

Minimum score: 0 points
Maximum score: 100 points

The higher the score, the higher the function.
Modified score: 0–100 points
Abbreviated score: 0–75 points

Validation

Outcomes validated against [1]

- Oxford shoulder score

Outcomes validated against [2]

- Oxford shoulder score
- Change in day-to-day life
- Improvement
- Success of operation
- SF-36

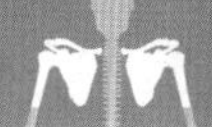

Validation (cont)

Outcomes validated against [3]
- DASH
- ASES
- SST

Patient population tested in	Validity	Reliability	Responsiveness
Patients with frozen shoulders (53 years; 52% male) [1]	- *	not tested	not tested
Patients who underwent rotator cuff surgery (57.8 years; 66% male) [2]	+/-	not tested	-
Patients who underwent open repair of supraspinatus and infraspinatus (55.3 years; 70% male) [3]	+	not tested	+
Patients with "abnormal" shoulders (Age NR; % male NR) [4]	not tested	+	not tested
Patients with shoulder dysfunction (49.2 years; 65% male) [5]	not tested	+	not tested
Patients who underwent decompression surgery for chronic impingement syndrome (62 years; 46% male) [6]	not tested	not tested	+

** + for the modified and abbreviated scores.*

Validation (cont)

Validation studies:

[1] Othman A, Taylor G (2004) Is the constant score reliable in assessing patients with frozen shoulder? 60 shoulders scored 3 years after manipulation under anaesthesia. Acta Orthop Scand; 75:114–116.
[2] Dawson J, Hill G, Fitzpatrick R, et al (2001) The benefits of using patient-based methods of assessment. Medium-term results of an observational study of shoulder surgery. J Bone Joint Surg Br; 83:877–882.
[3] Skutek M, Fremerey RW, Zeichen J, et al (2000) Outcome analysis following open rotator cuff repair. Early effectiveness validated using four different shoulder assessment scales. Arch Orthop Trauma Surg; 120:432–436.
[4] Constant CR, Murley AH (1987) A clinical method of functional assessment of the shoulder. Clin Orthop (214);160–164.
[5] Cook KF, Roddey TS, Olson SL, et al (2002) Reliability by surgical status of self-reported outcomes in patients who have shoulder pathologies. J Orthop Sports Phys Ther; 32:336–346.
[6] O'Connor DA, Chipchase LS, Tomlinson J, et al (1999) Arthroscopic subacromial decompression: responsiveness of disease-specific and health-related quality of life outcome measures. Arthroscopy; 15:836–840.

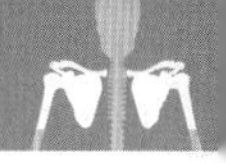

3. Constant-Murley functional assessment of the shoulder (1987)

Methodological evaluation ●●●○○○ (3/6)

		no score	0 points	1 point	points
Validity	Content validity	**not tested**	not valid	valid	-
Validity	Construct validity	not tested	not valid	**valid**	1
Validity	Criterion validity	not tested	**not valid**	valid	0
Reliability	Internal consistency	**not tested**	not consistent	consistent	-
Reliability	Reproducibility	not tested	not reproducible	**reproducible**	1
	Responsiveness	not tested	not responsive	**responsive**	1
				Subtotal	3

Clinical utility ●●●○ (3/4)

	0 points	1 point	2 points	points
Patient friendliness	limited	moderate	**strong**	2
Clinician friendliness	limited	**moderate**	strong	1
			Subtotal	3

Total (out of 10) ●●●●●●○○○○ **6**

4. Disabilities of the Arm, Shoulder and Hand (DASH) (1996)

Quick DASH see page 78.

Source: Hudak PL, Amadio PC, Bombardier C (1996) Development of an upper extremity outcome measure: the DASH (disabilities of the arm, shoulder and hand) [corrected]. The Upper Extremity Collaborative Group (UECG). Am J Ind Med; 29(6):602–608.

Other versions available: Chinese, Dutch, French, German, Hebrew, Italian, Norwegian, Spanish, Swedish, Taiwan Chinese, Turkish.
http://www.dash.iwh.on.ca

Content

Type Patient reported outcome
3 modules (one required, two optional)

Module 1: ability to perform (required)
Scale 6 subscales (30 items):

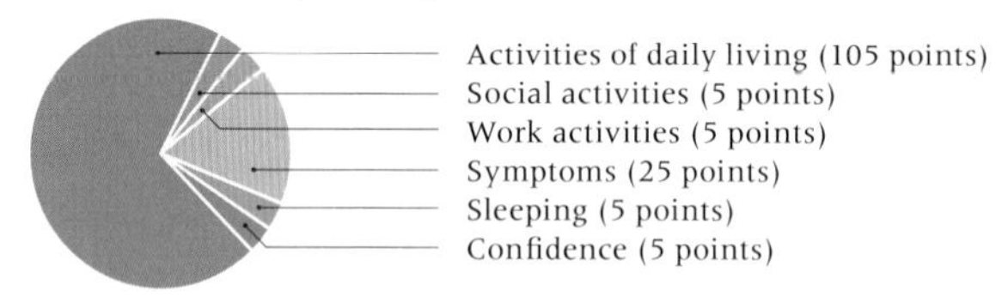

Module 2: ability to perform sports/performing arts (optional)
Scale
Sports/performing arts (20 points)

Module 3: ability to perform work (optional)
Scale
Work (20 points)

Interpretation
Each module is scored separately.

Normalized to 100:
[(Sum of responses / number of completed responses) - 1] × 25 = DASH score

Minimum score: 0 points
Maximum score: 100 points

The higher the score, the lower the function.

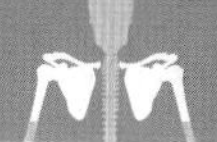

Validation

Outcomes validated against [1]
- SF-36

Outcomes validated against [2]
- SPADI
- Brigham (carpal tunnel) questionnaire
- VAS of pain, function, and ability to work

Outcomes validated against [3]
- Patient perception of change

Outcomes validated against [4]
- Number of actively inflamed joints
- Grip strength

Outcomes validated against [5]
- Constant-Murley shoulder score

Outcomes validated against [6]
- SF-12

Outcomes validated against [7]
- SF-36
- Health Assement Questionnaire (HAQ)
- Numeric pain rating scale
- Range of motion

Outcomes validated against [8]
- SF-36

Outcomes validated against [9]
- Canadian Occupational Performance Measure (COPM)

Patient population tested in	Validity	Reliability	Responsiveness
Patients with shoulder, elbow, wrist or hand complaints (40 years; 44% male) [1]	+	+	not tested
Patients with wrist/hand or shoulder disorders (53.6 years; 43% male) [2]	+	not tested	+
Patients with upper-extremity conditions planned for surgery (52 years; 42% male) [3]	+	+	+
Patients with psoriatic arthritis (49.2 years; 56% male) [4]	+	not tested	not tested
Patients who underwent open repair of supraspinatus and infraspinatus (55.3 years; 70% male) [5]	+	not tested	not tested
Swedish speaking patients with upper extremity conditions (52 years; 43% male) [6]	+	not tested	not tested

Validation (cont)

Patient population tested in	Validity	Reliability	Responsiveness
German speaking patients with shoulder pain (58.7 years; 27% male) [7]	+	not tested	not tested
Italian speaking patients with overuse syndromes of the shoulder, elbow, and wrist (54 years; 55% male) [8]	+	not tested	not tested
Dutch speaking patients with unilateral disorder of the upper limb (41 years; 48% male) [9]	+	not tested	not tested

Validation studies:

[1] SooHoo NF, McDonald AP, Seiler JG 3rd, et al (2002) Evaluation of the construct validity of the DASH questionnaire by correlation to the SF-36. J Hand Surg [Am]; 27: 537–541.
[2] Beaton DE, Katz JN, Fossel AH, et al (2001) Measuring the whole or the parts? Validity, reliability, and responsiveness of the Disabilities of the Arm, Shoulder and Hand outcome measure in different regions of the upper extremity. J Hand Ther; 14:128–146.
[3] Gummesson C, Atroshi I., Ekdahl C (2003) The disabilities of the arm, shoulder and hand (DASH) outcome questionnaire: longitudinal construct validity and measuring self-rated health change after surgery. BMC Musculoskelet Disord; 4(1):11.
[4] Navsarikar A, Gladman DD, Husted JA, et al (1999) Validity assessment of the disabilities of arm, shoulder, and hand questionnaire (DASH) for patients with psoriatic arthritis. J Rheumatol; 26:2191–2194.
[5] Skutek M, Fremerey RW, Zeichen J, et al (2000) Outcome analysis following open rotator cuff repair. Early effectiveness validated using four different shoulder assessment scales. Arch Orthop Trauma Surg; 120:432–436.
[6] Atroshi I, Gummesson C, Andersson B, et al (2000) The disabilities of the arm, shoulder and hand (DASH) outcome questionnaire: reliability and validity of the Swedish version evaluated in 176 patients. Acta Orthop Scand; 71:613–618.
[7] Offenbacher M, Ewert T, Sangha O, et al (2003) Validation of a German version of the ‚Disabilities of Arm, Shoulder and Hand' questionnaire (DASH-G). Z Rheumatol; 62:168–177.
[8] Padua R, Padua L, Ceccarelli E, et al (2003) Italian version of the Disability of the Arm, Shoulder and Hand (DASH) questionnaire. Cross-cultural adaptation and validation. J Hand Surg [Br]; 28:179–186.
[9] Veehof MM, Sleegers EJ, van Veldhoven NH, et al (2002) Psychometric qualities of the Dutch language version of the Disabilities of the Arm, Shoulder, and Hand questionnaire (DASH-DLV). J Hand Ther; 15:347–354.

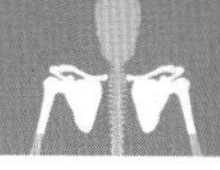

4. Disabilities of the Arm, Shoulder and Hand (DASH) (1996)

Methodological evaluation ●●●●●● (6/6)

		no score	0 points	1 point	points
Validity	Content validity	not tested	not valid	**valid**	1
	Construct validity	not tested	not valid	**valid**	1
	Criterion validity	not tested	not valid	**valid**	1
Reliability	Internal consistency	not tested	not consistent	**consistent**	1
	Reproducibility	not tested	not reproducible	**reproducible**	1
	Responsiveness	not tested	not responsive	**responsive**	1
				Subtotal	**6**

Clinical utility ●●○○ (2/4)

	0 points	1 point	2 points	points
Patient friendliness	**limited**	moderate	strong	0
Clinician friendliness	limited	moderate	**strong**	2
			Subtotal	**2**

Total (out of 10)	●●●●●●●●○○	**8**

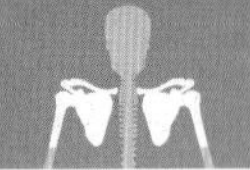

5. Flexilevel scale of Shoulder Function (FLEX-SF) (2003)

Source: Cook KF, Roddey TS, Gartsman GM, Olson SL (2003) Development and psychometric evaluation of the Flexilevel Scale of Shoulder Function. Med Care; 41: 823–835.

Content

Type Patient reported outcome
Scale 3 subscales (15 items):

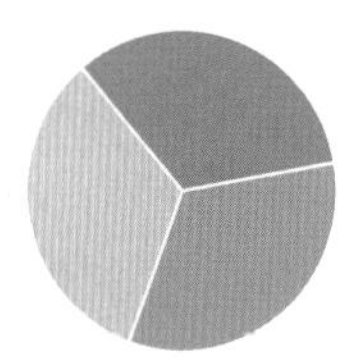

Patient completes one of three 'testlets' (easy, medium, hard) based on their response to a screening question.
The purpose of the testlets is to make the instrument adaptive and flexible for multiple patient populations.

Each 'testlet' contains 15 items: Likert scale for each item (5 choices; 0–4 points each).

Interpretation

Raw score: summing item responses.

Minimum: 0 points
Maximum: 60 points

FLEX-SF score: calibrated and linearly transformed.

The higher the score, the higher the function.

Validation

Outcomes validated against

- SF-12
- ASES

Patient population tested in	Validity	Reliability	Responsiveness
Patients with shoulder complaints (52 years; 53% male)	+	+	+

Validation study:

Cook KF, Roddey TS, Gartsman GM, Olson SL (2003) Development and psychometric evaluation of the Flexilevel Scale of Shoulder Function. Med Care, 41: 823–835.

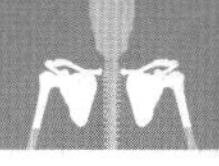

Methodological evaluation ●●●●●○ (5/6)

		no score	0 points	1 point	points
Validity	Content validity	not tested	not valid	valid	1
	Construct validity	not tested	not valid	valid	1
	Criterion validity	not tested	not valid	valid	-
Reliability	Internal consistency	not tested	not consistent	consistent	1
	Reproducibility	not tested	not reproducible	reproducible	1
	Responsiveness	not tested	not responsive	responsive	1
				Subtotal	**5**

Clinical utility ●●●● (4/4)

	0 points	1 point	2 points	points
Patient friendliness	limited	moderate	strong	2
Clinician friendliness	limited	moderate	strong	2
			Subtotal	**4**

Total (out of 10) ●●●●●●●●●○ **9**

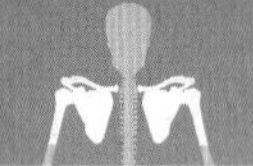

6. Herscovici shoulder scale (1992)

Source: Herscovici D Jr, Fiennes AG, Allgower M, Ruedi TP (1992) The floating shoulder: ipsilateral clavicle and scapular neck fractures. J Bone Joint Surg Br; 74: 362–364.

Content

Type Clinician based outcome
Scale 4 subscales (4 items):

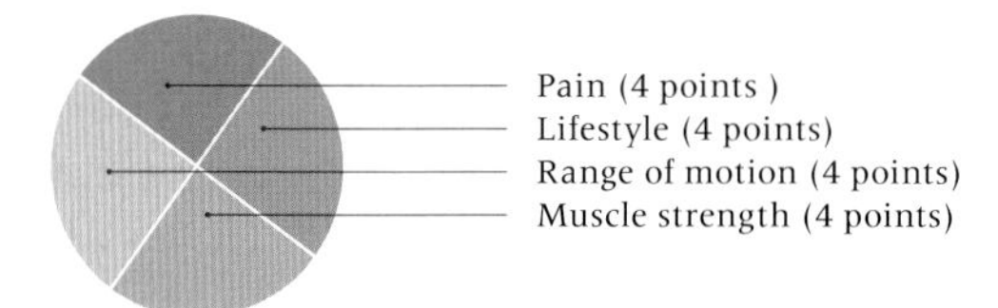

Interpretation

Excellent: 13–16 points
Good: 9–12 points
Fair: 5–9 points
Poor: < 4 points

Validation

No validation studies were identified.

Patient population tested in	Validity	Reliability	Responsiveness
Not applicable			

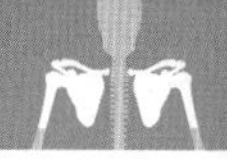

Methodological evaluation ○○○○○○ (0/6)

		no score	0 points	1 point	points
Validity	Content validity	not tested	not valid	valid	-
	Construct validity	not tested	not valid	valid	-
	Criterion validity	not tested	not valid	valid	-
Reliability	Internal consistency	not tested	not consistent	consistent	-
	Reproducibility	not tested	not reproducible	reproducible	-
	Responsiveness	not tested	not responsive	responsive	-
				Subtotal	-

Clinical utility ●●●● (4/4)

	0 points	1 point	2 points	points
Patient friendliness	limited	moderate	strong	2
Clinician friendliness	limited	moderate	strong	2
			Subtotal	**4**

Total (out of 10) ●●●●○○○○○○ **4**

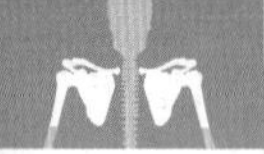

7. Hospital for Special Surgery shoulder assessment (HSS) (1982)

Source: Warren RF, Ranawat CS, I. AE (1982) Total shoulder replacement. Indications and results of the Neer non-constrained prosthesis. In: AAOS Symposium on Total Joint Replacement of the Upper Extremity.
Edited by I. AE. St Louis; CV Mosby, pp. 56–67.

Content

Type Clinician based outcome
Scale 4 subscales (7 items):

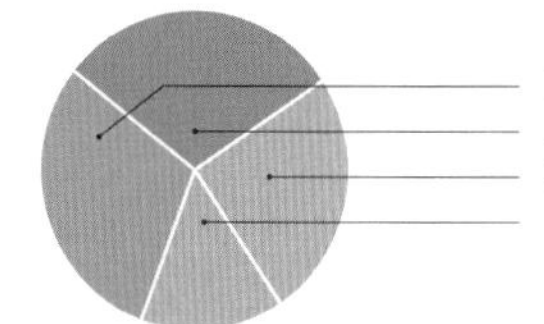

Interpretation
Minimum score: 0 points
Maximum score: 100 points

Validation

No validation studies were identified.

Patient population tested in	Validity	Reliability	Responsiveness
Not applicable			

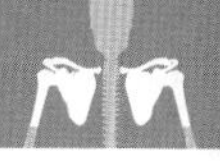

7. Hospital for Special Surgery shoulder assessment (HSS) (1982)

Methodological evaluation ○○○○○○ (0/6)

		no score	0 points	1 point	points
Validity	Content validity	not tested	not valid	valid	-
	Construct validity	not tested	not valid	valid	-
	Criterion validity	not tested	not valid	valid	-
Reliability	Internal consistency	not tested	not consistent	consistent	-
	Reproducibility	not tested	not reproducible	reproducible	-
	Responsiveness	not tested	not responsive	responsive	-
				Subtotal	-

Clinical utility ●●●○ (3/4)

	0 points	1 point	2 points	points
Patient friendliness	limited	moderate	strong	2
Clinician friendliness	limited	moderate	strong	1
			Subtotal	3

Total (out of 10) ●●●○○○○○○○ **3**

8. Imatani shoulder score (1975)

Source: Imatani RJ, Hanlon JJ, Cady GW (1975) Acute, complete acromioclavicular separation.
J Bone Joint Surg Am; 57:328–332.

Content

Type Clinician based outcome
Scale 3 subscales (7 items):

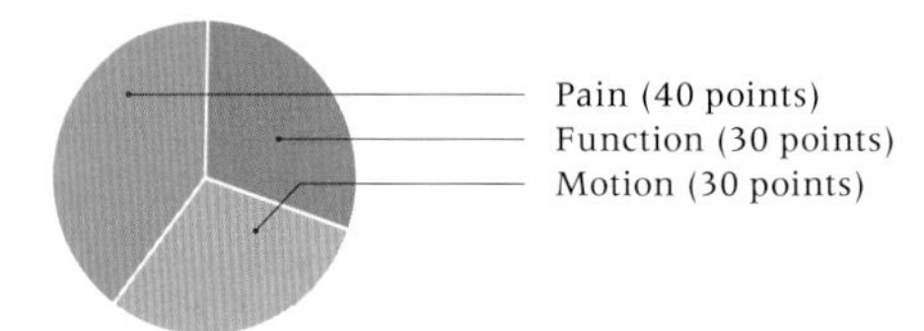

Interpretation
Excellent: 90–100 points
Good: 80–89 points
Fair: 70–79 points
Poor: < 70 points

Validation

No validation studies were identified.

Patient population tested in	Validity	Reliability	Responsiveness
Not applicable			

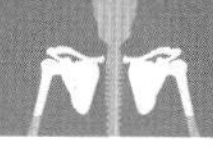

8. Imatani shoulder score (1975)

Methodological evaluation

○○○○○○ (0/6)

		no score	0 points	1 point	points
Validity	Content validity	not tested	not valid	valid	-
	Construct validity	not tested	not valid	valid	-
	Criterion validity	not tested	not valid	valid	-
Reliability	Internal consistency	not tested	not consistent	consistent	-
	Reproducibility	not tested	not reproducible	reproducible	-
	Responsiveness	not tested	not responsive	responsive	-
				Subtotal	-

Clinical utility

●●●● (4/4)

	0 points	1 point	2 points	points
Patient friendliness	limited	moderate	strong	2
Clinician friendliness	limited	moderate	strong	2
			Subtotal	**4**

Total (out of 10) ●●●●○○○○○○ **4**

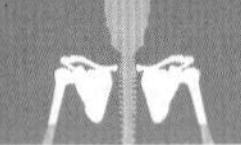

9. L'Insalata shoulder rating system (1997)

Source: L'Insalata JC, Warren RF, Cohen SB, Altchek DW, Peterson MG (1997) A self-administered questionnaire for assessment of symptoms and function of the shoulder.
J Bone Joint Surg Am; 79:738–748.

Content

Type Patient reported outcome
Scale 6 subscales (21 items):

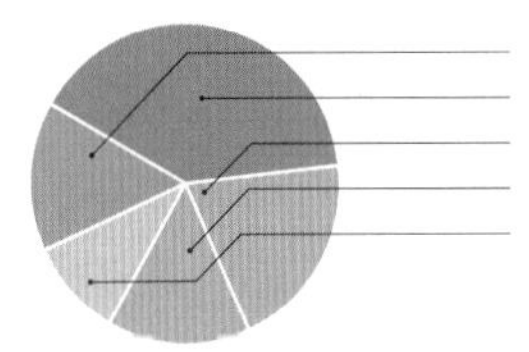

Global assessment (15 points)
Pain (40 points)
Activities of daily living (20 points)
Recreational and athletic activities (15 points)
Work (10 points)
Satisfaction (poor to excellent; not included in total score)

A final nongraded domain allows the patient to select two areas in which he/she believes improvement is most important.

Interpretation

Each domain is scored separately by averaging the scores of completed questions and multiplying by 2.

Minimum score: 17 points   Maximum score: 100 points

Validation

Outcomes validated against

- Arthritis Impact Measurement Scales 2
- Global assessment domain and each domain category (pain, daily function, recreational and athletic function, and work) were correlated with a single question assessing their satisfaction in each area.

Patient population tested in	Validity	Reliability	Responsiveness
Patients with shoulder complaints (40 years; 73% male)	+	+	+

Validation study:

L'Insalata JC, Warren RF, Cohen SB, et al (1997) A self-administered questionnaire for assessment of symptoms and function of the shoulder. J Bone Joint Surg Am; 79:738–748.

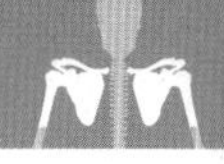

Methodological evaluation ●●●●●○ (5/6)

		no score	0 points	1 point	points
Validity	Content validity	not tested	not valid	**valid**	1
	Construct validity	not tested	not valid	**valid**	1
	Criterion validity	**not tested**	not valid	valid	-
Reliability	Internal consistency	not tested	not consistent	**consistent**	1
	Reproducibility	not tested	not reproducible	**reproducible**	1
	Responsiveness	not tested	not responsive	**responsive**	1
				Subtotal	**5**

Clinical utility ●●○○ (2/4)

	0 points	1 point	2 points	points
Patient friendliness	**limited**	moderate	strong	0
Clinician friendliness	limited	moderate	**strong**	2
			Subtotal	**2**

Total (out of 10) ●●●●●●●○○○ **7**

10. Neer shoulder score (1970)

Source: Neer CS 2nd (1970) Displaced proximal humeral fractures. I. Classification and evaluation. J Bone Joint Surg Am; 52:3–10.

Content

Type Clinician based outcome
Scale 4 subscales (18 items):

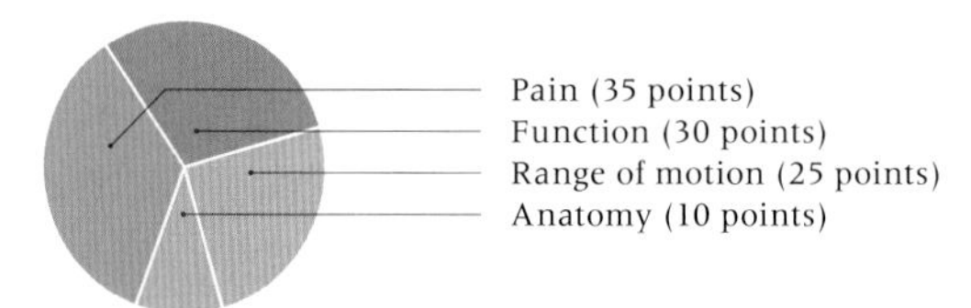

Interpretation
Excellent: 90–100 points
Satisfactory: 80–89 points
Unsatisfactory: 70–79 points
Failure: < 70 points

Validation

No validation studies were identified.

Patient population tested in	Validity	Reliability	Responsiveness
Not applicable			

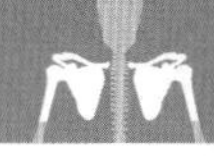

Methodological evaluation ○○○○○○ (0/6)

		no score	0 points	1 point	points
Validity	Content validity	not tested	not valid	valid	-
	Construct validity	not tested	not valid	valid	-
	Criterion validity	not tested	not valid	valid	-
Reliability	Internal consistency	not tested	not consistent	consistent	-
	Reproducibility	not tested	not reproducible	reproducible	-
	Responsiveness	not tested	not responsive	responsive	-
				Subtotal	-

Clinical utility ●●●○ (3/4)

	0 points	1 point	2 points	points
Patient friendliness	limited	moderate	strong	2
Clinician friendliness	limited	moderate	strong	1
			Subtotal	**3**

Total (out of 10) ●●●○○○○○○○ **3**

11. Oxford shoulder score (1996)

Source: Dawson J, Fitzpatrick R, Carr A (1996) Questionnaire on the perceptions of patients about shoulder surgery.
J Bone Joint Surg Br; 78:593–600.

Content

Type Patient reported outcome
Scale 2 subscales (12 items):

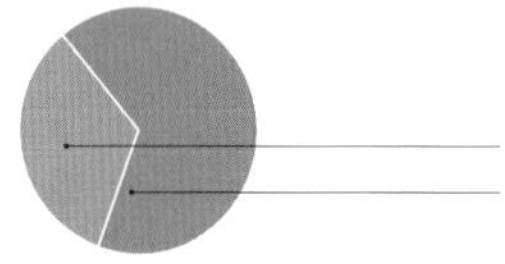

5-point Likert scale divided into the following general areas:
Pain (20 points)
Activities of daily living (40 points)

Interpretation
Minimum score: 12 points; maximum score: 60 points
The higher the score, the lower the function.

Validation

Outcomes validated against [1]
- Constant-Murley shoulder score
- SF-36
- Health Assessment Questionnaire
- Change in day-to-day life
- Improvement
- Success of operation

Outcomes validated against [2]
- Constant-Murley shoulder score
- SF-36

Outcomes validated against [3]
- Constant-Murley shoulder score

Patient population tested in	Validity	Reliability	Responsiveness
Patients with chronic shoulder complaints (57.4 years; 55% male) [1]	+	+	+
Patients who underwent rotator cuff surgery (57.8 years; 66% male) [2]	+	not tested	+
Patients with frozen shoulders (53 years; 52% male) [3]	+	not tested	not tested

Validation studies:

[1] Dawson J, Fitzpatrick R, Carr A (1996) Questionnaire on the perceptions of patients about shoulder surgery. J Bone Joint Surg Br; 78:593–600.
[2] Dawson J, Hill G, Fitzpatrick R, et al (2001) The benefits of using patient-based methods of assessment. Medium-term results of an observational study of shoulder surgery. J Bone Joint Surg Br; 83:877–882.
[3] Othman A, Taylor G (2004) Is the constant score reliable in assessing patients with frozen shoulder? 60 shoulders scored 3 years after manipulation under anaesthesia. Acta Orthop Scand; 75:114–116.

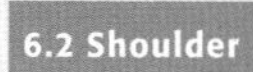

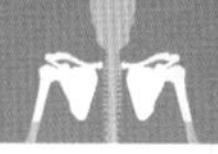

Methodological evaluation

●●●●●● (6/6)

		no score	0 points	1 point	points
Validity	Content validity	not tested	not valid	valid	1
	Construct validity	not tested	not valid	valid	1
	Criterion validity	not tested	not valid	valid	1
Reliability	Internal consistency	not tested	not consistent	consistent	1
	Reproducibility	not tested	not reproducible	reproducible	1
	Responsiveness	not tested	not responsive	responsive	1
				Subtotal	**6**

Clinical utility

●●●○ (3/4)

	0 points	1 point	2 points	points
Patient friendliness	limited	moderate	strong	1
Clinician friendliness	limited	moderate	strong	2
			Subtotal	**3**

Total (out of 10) ●●●●●●●●●○ **9**

12. Quick DASH (1996)

Source: King GJ, Richards RR, Zuckerman JD, Blasier R, Dillman C, Friedman RJ, Gartsman GM, Iannotti JP, Murnahan JP, Mow VC, Woo SL (1999) A standardized method for assessment of elbow function. Research Committee, American Shoulder and Elbow Surgeons. J Shoulder Elbow Surg; 8:351–354.

Content

3 modules
Module 1: ability to perform (required)
Scale 5 subscales (11 items):

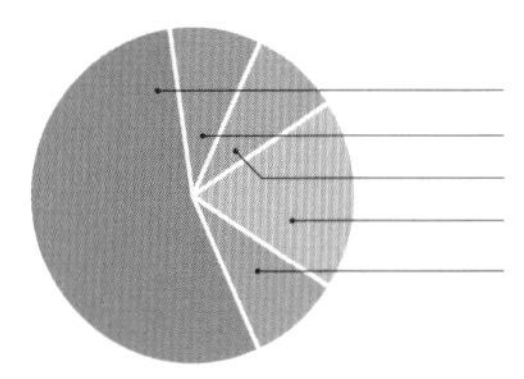

Module 2: ability to perform sports/performing arts (optional)
Scale
Sports/performing arts (20 points)

Module 3: ability to perform work (optional)
Scale
Work (20 points)

Interpretation
Each module is scored separately.

Normalized to 100:
[(Sum of responses / number of completed responses) – 1] × 25 = Quick DASH score

Minimum score: 0 points
Maximum score: 100 points

The higher the score, the lower the function.

Validation

No validation studies were identified.

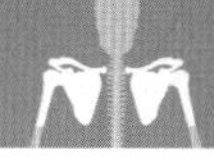

Methodological evaluation ○○○○○○ (0/6)

		no score	0 points	1 point	points
Validity	Content validity	not tested	not valid	valid	-
	Construct validity	not tested	not valid	valid	-
	Criterion validity	not tested	not valid	valid	-
Reliability	Internal consistency	not tested	not consistent	consistent	-
	Reproducibility	not tested	not reproducible	reproducible	-
	Responsiveness	not tested	not responsive	responsive	-
				Subtotal	-

Clinical utility ●●●○ (3/4)

	0 points	1 point	2 points	points
Patient friendliness	limited	moderate	strong	1
Clinician friendliness	limited	moderate	strong	2
			Subtotal	3

Total (out of 10) ●●●○○○○○○○ **3**

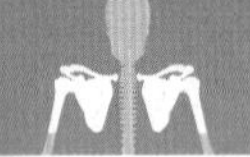

13. Rotator Cuff Quality of Life measure (RC-QOL) (2000)

Source: Hollinshead RM, Mohtadi NG, Vande Guchte RA, Wadey VM (2000) Two 6-year follow-up studies of large and massive rotator cuff tears: comparison of outcome measures.
J Shoulder Elbow Surg; 9:373–381.

Content

Type Patient reported outcome
Scale 5 subscales (34 items):

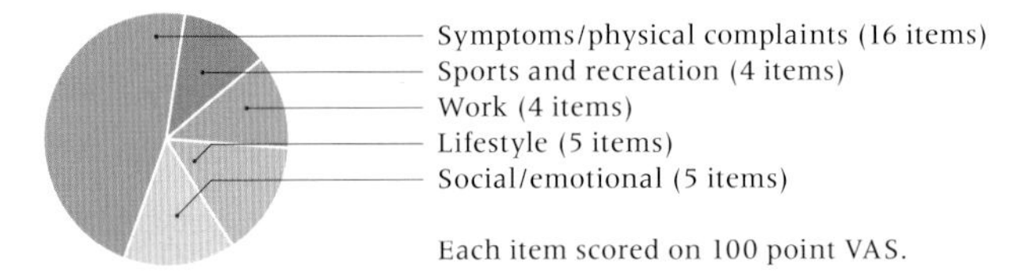

Interpretation

Average of all items = RC-QOL score.
The higher the score, the higher the function.

Validation

Outcomes validated against

- SF-36
- ASES
- Functional Shoulder Elevation Test

Patient population tested in	Validity	Reliability	Responsiveness
Patients who underwent surgical treatment for rotator cuff tear. (63 years; 69% male)	+	+	not tested

Validation study:

Hollinshead RM, Mohtadi NG, Vande Guchte RA, et al (2000) Two 6-year follow-up studies of large and massive rotator cuff tears: comparison of outcome measures. J Shoulder Elbow Surg; 9:373–381.

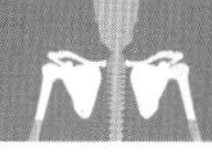

Methodological evaluation

●●●○○○ (3/6)

		no score	0 points	1 point	points
Validity	Content validity	not tested	not valid	**valid**	1
	Construct validity	not tested	not valid	**valid**	1
	Criterion validity	**not tested**	not valid	valid	-
Reliability	Internal consistency	**not tested**	not consistent	consistent	-
	Reproducibility	not tested	not reproducible	**reproducible**	1
	Responsiveness	**not tested**	not responsive	responsive	-
				Subtotal	**3**

Clinical utility

●●○○ (2/4)

	0 points	1 point	2 points	points
Patient friendliness	**limited**	moderate	strong	0
Clinician friendliness	limited	moderate	**strong**	2
			Subtotal	**2**

Total (out of 10) ●●●●●○○○○○ **5**

14. Rowe shoulder score (also known as rating sheet for Bankart repair) (1978)

Source: Rowe CR, Patel D, Southmayd WW (1978) The Bankart procedure: a long-term end-result study.
J Bone Joint Surg Am; 60:1–16.

Content

Type Clinician based outcome
Scale 3 subscales (3 items):

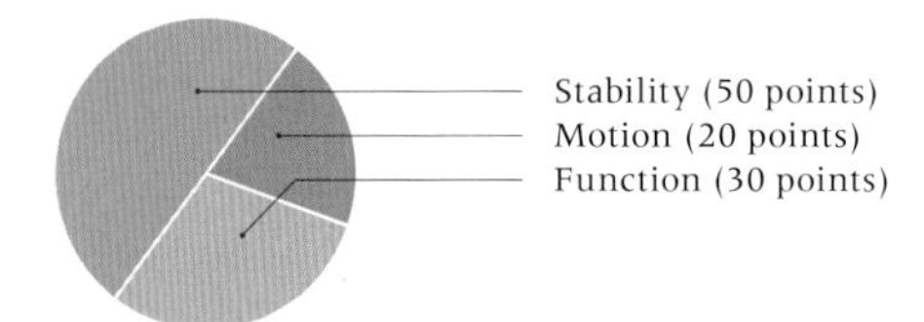

Interpretation
Excellent: 90–100 points
Good: 75–89 points
Fair: 51–74 points
Poor: < 51 points

Validation

Outcomes validated against
- ASES
- SANE

Patient population tested in	Validity	Reliability	Responsiveness
Patients who underwent shoulder surgery for instability or significant AC separations (20 years; 90% male)	+	not tested	+

Validation study:
Williams GN, Gangel TJ, Arciero RA, et al (1999) Comparison of the Single Assessment Numeric Evaluation method and two shoulder rating scales. Outcomes measures after shoulder surgery. Am J Sports Med; 27:214–221.

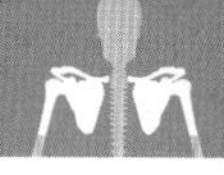

14. Rowe shoulder score (also known as rating sheet for Bankart repair) (1978)

Methodological evaluation ●●○○○○ (2/6)

		no score	0 points	1 point	points
Validity	Content validity	not tested	not valid	valid	-
	Construct validity	not tested	not valid	valid	-
	Criterion validity	not tested	not valid	valid	1
Reliability	Internal consistency	not tested	not consistent	consistent	-
	Reproducibility	not tested	not reproducible	reproducible	-
	Responsiveness	not tested	not responsive	responsive	1
				Subtotal	2

Clinical utility ●●●● (4/4)

	0 points	1 point	2 points	points
Patient friendliness	limited	moderate	strong	2
Clinician friendliness	limited	moderate	strong	2
			Subtotal	4

Total (out of 10) ●●●●●●○○○○ **6**

15. Shoulder disability questionnaire–Croft (1994)

Source: Croft P, Pope D, Zonca M, O'Neill T, Silman A (1994) Measurement of shoulder related disability: results of a validation study.
Ann Rheum Dis; 53:525–528.

Content

Type Patient reported outcome

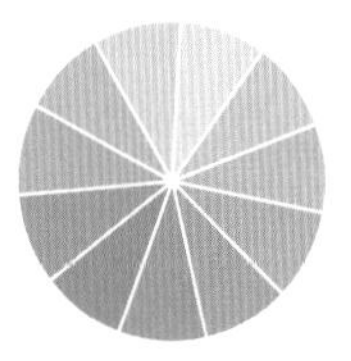

22 items covering 11 disability categories in the following areas:
- Activities of daily living
- Recreational activities
- Psychosocial issues
- Pain and stiffness

Interpretation

Minimum score: 0 points
Maximum score: 100 points
Score = (number of affirmative answers / number of applicable items) × 100

The higher the score, the lower the function.

Validation

Outcomes validated against

- Shoulder range of motion
- Shoulder power

Patient population tested in	Validity	Reliability	Responsiveness
Subjects in the community with shoulder pain (65 years; 38% male) Patients attending primary care for shoulder pain (51 years; 48% male)	+	not tested	not tested

Validation study:

Croft P, Pope D, Zonca M, et al (1994) Measurement of shoulder related disability: results of a validation study. Ann Rheum Dis; 53:525–528.

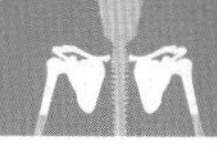

Methodological evaluation ●●○○○○ (2/6)

		no score	0 points	1 point	points
Validity	Content validity	not tested	not valid	**valid**	1
	Construct validity	not tested	not valid	**valid**	1
	Criterion validity	**not tested**	not valid	valid	-
Reliability	Internal consistency	**not tested**	not consistent	consistent	-
	Reproducibility	**not tested**	not reproducible	reproducible	-
	Responsiveness	**not tested**	not responsive	responsive	-
				Subtotal	**2**

Clinical utility ●●○○ (2/4)

	0 points	1 point	2 points	points
Patient friendliness	**limited**	moderate	strong	0
Clinician friendliness	limited	moderate	**strong**	2
			Subtotal	**2**

Total (out of 10) ●●●●○○○○○○ **4**

16. Shoulder disability questionnaire–van der Heijden (2000)

Source: van der Heijden GJ, Leffers P, Bouter LM (2000) Shoulder disability questionnaire design and responsiveness of a functional status measure.
J Clin Epidemiol; 53:29–38.

Content

Type Patient reported outcome

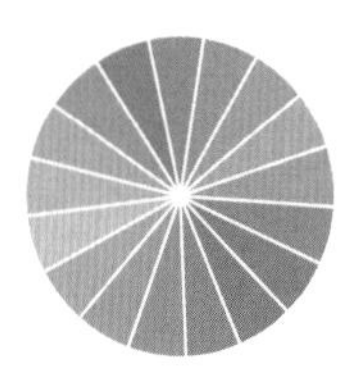

16 items covering common situations which may induce shoulder complaints. Possible answers include yes, no or not applicable.

Interpretation
Minimum score: 0 points
Maximum score: 100 points
Score = (number of affirmative answers / number of applicable items) × 100
The higher the score, the lower the function.

Validation

Not applicable.

Patient population tested in	Validity	Reliability	Responsiveness
Patients with soft tissue shoulder disorders (51 years; 49% male) [1] [2]	not tested	not tested	+
Patients with shoulder disorders presenting to primary care (49.6 years; 44% male) [2]	not tested	not tested	+

Validation studies:

[1] van der Heijden GJ, Leffers P, Bouter LM (2000) Shoulder disability questionnaire design and responsiveness of a functional status measure. J Clin Epidemiol; 53:29–38.
[2] van der Windt DA, van der Heijden GJ, de Winter AF, et al (1998) The responsiveness of the Shoulder Disability Questionnaire. Ann Rheum Dis; 57: 82–87.

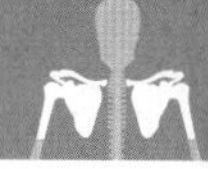

16. Shoulder disability questionnaire–van der Heijden (2000)

Methodological evaluation ●○○○○○ (1/6)

		no score	0 points	1 point	points
Validity	Content validity	not tested	not valid	valid	-
	Construct validity	not tested	not valid	valid	-
	Criterion validity	not tested	not valid	valid	-
Reliability	Internal consistency	not tested	not consistent	consistent	-
	Reproducibility	not tested	not reproducible	reproducible	-
	Responsiveness	not tested	not responsive	responsive	1
				Subtotal	**1**

Clinical utility ●●●○ (3/4)

	0 points	1 point	2 points	points
Patient friendliness	limited	moderate	strong	1
Clinician friendliness	limited	moderate	strong	2
			Subtotal	**3**

Total (out of 10) ●●●●○○○○○○ **4**

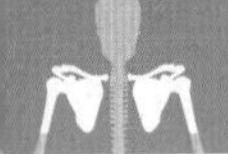

17. Shoulder instability questionnaire (1999)

Source: Dawson J, Fitzpatrick R, Carr A (1999) The assessment of shoulder instability. The development and validation of a questionnaire.
J Bone Joint Surg Br; 81:420–426.

Content

Type Patient reported outcome
Scale 5 subscales (12 items):

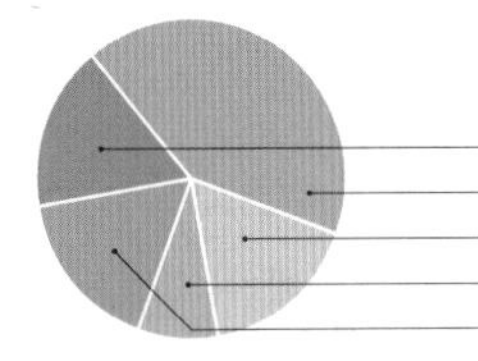

5-point Likert scale divided into the following general areas:
Instability (10 points)
Activities of daily living (25 points)
Pain (10 points)
Work (5 points)
Social/recreation (10 points)

Interpretation

Minimum score: 12 points
Maximum score: 60 points

The higher the score, the lower the function.

Validation

Outcomes validated against

- Rowe shoulder score
- SF-36
- Constant-Murley shoulder score

Patient population tested in	Validity	Reliability	Responsiveness
Patients with instability of the shoulder (26.3 years; 61% male)	+	+	+

Validation study:
Dawson J, Fitzpatrick R, Carr A (1999) The assessment of shoulder instability. The development and validation of a questionnaire.
J Bone Joint Surg Br; 81:420–426.

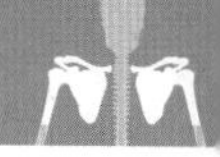

Methodological evaluation

●●●●●○ (5/6)

		no score	0 points	1 point	points
Validity	Content validity	not tested	not valid	**valid**	1
	Construct validity	not tested	not valid	**valid**	1
	Criterion validity	**not tested**	not valid	valid	-
Reliability	Internal consistency	not tested	not consistent	**consistent**	1
	Reproducibility	not tested	not reproducible	**reproducible**	1
	Responsiveness	not tested	not responsive	**responsive**	1
				Subtotal	**5**

Clinical utility

●●●○ (3/4)

	0 points	1 point	2 points	points
Patient friendliness	limited	**moderate**	strong	1
Clinician friendliness	limited	moderate	**strong**	2
			Subtotal	**3**

Total (out of 10)  **8**

18. Shoulder Pain and Disability Index (SPADI) (1991)

Source: O'Connor DA, Chipchase LS, Tomlinson J, et al (1999) Arthroscopic subacromial decompression: responsiveness of disease-specific and health-related quality of life outcome measures.
Arthroscopy; 15:836–840.

Content

Type Patient reported outcome
Scale 2 subscales (13 items):

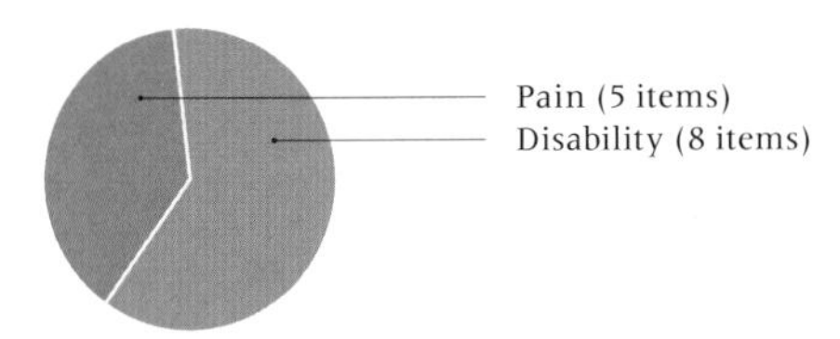

All items rated by using a VAS divided into 12 segments. A number ranging from 0 to 11 was assigned to each item.

Subscale score = (adding item scores for that subscale / maximum score possible for the items deemed applicable by the subject) × 100

Interpretation
Minimum score: 0 points
Maximum score: 100 points

Total SPADI score = average of pain and disability subscale scores

The higher the score, the lower the function.

Validation

Outcomes validated against [1]
- Shoulder range of motion

Outcomes validated against [2]
- Subjective shoulder rating scale
- ASES
- SST
- Shoulder Severity Index
- SF-36

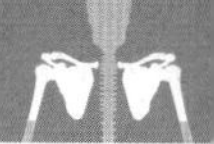

Validation (cont)

Outcomes validated against [3]

- SF-20
- Health Assessment Questionnaire

Outcomes validated against [4]

- Sickness impact profile

Outcomes validated against [5]

- UCLA End-Result score

Patient population tested in	Validity	Reliability	Responsiveness
Patients with shoulder pain (58 years; 100% male) [1]	+	+	+
Patients who underwent rotator cuff surgery or total shoulder arthroplasty (55 years; 59% male) [2]	not tested	not tested	+
Patients expected to be stable in their shoulder function (48 years; 45% male) [2]	not tested	+	not tested
Patients with shoulder discomfort (60 years; 98% male) [3]	+	not tested	+
Patients referred to outpatient physical therapy for shoulder pain (44.8 years; 64.8% male) [4]	+	not tested	+
Patients with shoulder disorders (47 years; 58% male) [5]	+	+	not tested
Patients with shoulder dysfunction (49.2 years; 65% male) [6]	not tested	+	not tested

Validation (cont)

Validation studies:

[1] Roach KE, Budiman-Mak E, Songsiridej N, et al (1991) Development of a shoulder pain and disability index. Arthritis Care Res; 4:143–149.
[2] Beaton D., Richards RR (1998) Assessing the reliability and responsiveness of 5 shoulder questionnaires. J Shoulder Elbow Surg; 7: 565–572.
[3] Williams JW Jr, Holleman DR Jr, Simel DL (1995) Measuring shoulder function with the Shoulder Pain and Disability Index. J Rheumatol; 22: 727–732.
[4] Heald SL, Riddle DL, Lamb RL (1997) The shoulder pain and disability index: the construct validity and responsiveness of a region-specific disability measure. Phys Ther; 77:1079–1089.
[5] Roddey TS, Olson SL, Cook KF, et al (2000) Comparison of the University of California-Los Angeles Shoulder Scale and the Simple Shoulder Test with the shoulder pain and disability index: single-administration reliability and validity. Phys Ther; 80:759–768.
[6] Cook KF, Roddey TS, Olson SL, et al (2002) Reliability by surgical status of self-reported outcomes in patients who have shoulder pathologies. J Orthop Sports Phys Ther; 32:336–346.

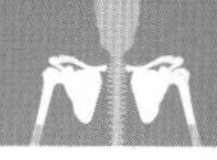

18. Shoulder Pain and Disability Index (SPADI) (1991)

Methodological evaluation ●●●●●● (6/6)

		no score	0 points	1 point	points
Validity	Content validity	not tested	not valid	valid	1
	Construct validity	not tested	not valid	valid	1
	Criterion validity	not tested	not valid	valid	1
Reliability	Internal consistency	not tested	not consistent	consistent	1
	Reproducibility	not tested	not reproducible	reproducible	1
	Responsiveness	not tested	not responsive	responsive	1
				Subtotal	**6**

Clinical utility ●●●○ (3/4)

	0 points	1 point	2 points	points
Patient friendliness	limited	moderate	strong	1
Clinician friendliness	limited	moderate	strong	2
			Subtotal	**3**

Total (out of 10) ●●●●●●●●●○ **9**

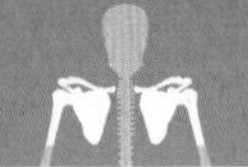

19. Shoulder pain score (1996)

Source: Winters JC, Sobel JS, Groenier KH, Arendzen JH, Meyboom-De Jong B (1996) A shoulder pain score: a comprehensive questionnaire for assessing pain in patients with shoulder complaints. Scand J Rehabil Med; 28:163–167.

Content

Type Patient reported outcome
Scale 7 items:

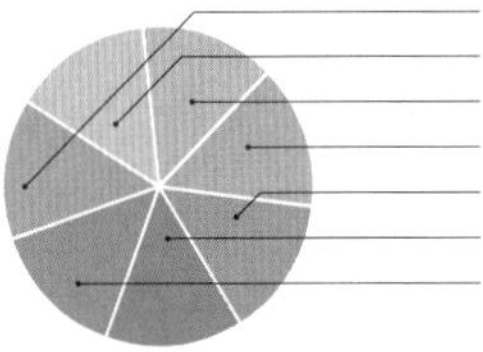

- Pain at rest (4 points)
- Pain in motion (4 points)
- Nightly pain (4 points)
- Sleeping problems caused by pain (4 points)
- Incapability of lying on the painful side (4 points)
- Degree of radiation (4 points)
- NRS-101 Pain Scale (4 points)

Likert scale for each item (4 choices). NRS-101 converted to a 4-point scale.

Interpretation

Minimum score: 7 points
Maximum score: 28 points
The higher the score, the lower the function.

Validation

Not applicable. Only content validity was assessed.

Patient population tested in	Validity	Reliability	Responsiveness
Patients with shoulder pain/ complaints (47.3 years; 42% male)	+	+	not tested

Validation study:
Winters JC, Sobel JS, Groenier KH, et al (1996) A shoulder pain score: a comprehensive questionnaire for assessing pain in patients with shoulder complaints. Scand J Rehabil Med; 28:163–167.

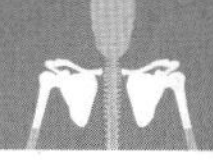

Methodological evaluation

●●○○○○ (2/6)

		no score	0 points	1 point	points
Validity	Content validity	not tested	not valid	**valid**	1
	Construct validity	**not tested**	not valid	valid	-
	Criterion validity	**not tested**	not valid	valid	-
Reliability	Internal consistency	not tested	not consistent	**consistent**	1
	Reproducibility	**not tested**	not reproducible	reproducible	-
	Responsiveness	**not tested**	not responsive	responsive	-
				Subtotal	**2**

Clinical utility

●●●● (4/4)

	0 points	1 point	2 points	points
Patient friendliness	limited	moderate	**strong**	2
Clinician friendliness	limited	moderate	**strong**	2
			Subtotal	**4**

Total (out of 10) ●●●●●●○○○○ **6**

20. Simple Shoulder Test (SST) (1993)

Source: Lippitt SB, H. D, Matsen FAI (1993) A practical tool for the evaluation of function: the simple shoulder test. In: The shoulder: a balance of mobility and stability.
Edited by F. F, Matsen FA, Hawkins RJ; Rosemont, IL: The American Academy of Orthopedic Surgeons,
pp. 501–518.

Content

Type Patient reported outcome
Scale 12 items:

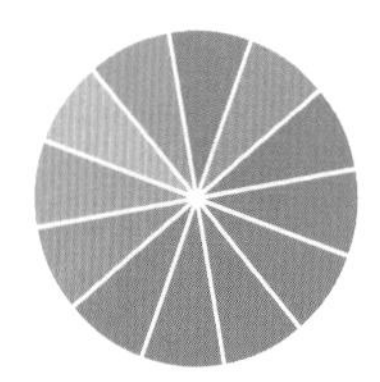

12 yes or no questions concerning the ability to perform 12 activities of daily living.

Interpretation

Minimum score: 0 points; maximum score: 100 points
Reported as a percentage of questions answered in the affirmative.
The higher the score, the higher the function.

Validation

Outcomes validated against [1]

- Subjective shoulder rating scale
- SPADI
- Modified-American Shoulder and Elbow Surgeons form
- Shoulder Severity Index
- SF-36

Outcomes validated against [2]

- Constant-Murley shoulder score

Outcomes validated against [3]

- UCLA End-Result score
- SPADI

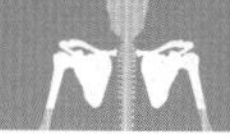

Validation (cont)

Patient population tested in	Validity	Reliability	Responsiveness
Patients who underwent rotator cuff surgery or total shoulder arthroplasty (55 years; 59% male) [1]	not tested	not tested	+
Patients expected to be stable in their shoulder function (48 years; 45% male) [1]	not tested	+	not tested
Patients with combined tears of supraspinatus and infraspinatus (55.3 years; 70% male) [2]	+	not tested	not tested
Patients with shoulder disorders (47 years; 58% male) [3]	+	+	not tested

Validation studies:

[1] Beaton D., Richards RR (1998) Assessing the reliability and responsiveness of 5 shoulder questionnaires. J Shoulder Elbow Surg; 7: 565–572.

[2] Skutek M, Fremerey RW, Zeichen J, et al (2000) Outcome analysis following open rotator cuff repair. Early effectiveness validated using four different shoulder assessment scales. Arch Orthop Trauma Surg; 120: 432–436.

[3] Roddey TS, Olson SL, Cook KF, et al (2000) Comparison of the University of California-Los Angeles Shoulder Scale and the Simple Shoulder Test with the shoulder pain and disability index: single-administration reliability and validity. Phys Ther; 80:759–768.

20. Simple Shoulder Test (SST) (1993)

Details see previous pages.

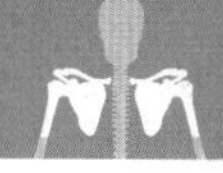

Methodological evaluation ●●●●●○ (5/6)

		no score	0 points	1 point	points
Validity	Content validity	not tested	not valid	valid	-
	Construct validity	not tested	not valid	valid	1
	Criterion validity	not tested	not valid	valid	1
Reliability	Internal consistency	not tested	not consistent	consistent	1
	Reproducibility	not tested	not reproducible	reproducible	1
	Responsiveness	not tested	not responsive	responsive	1
				Subtotal	**5**

Clinical utility ●●●○ (3/4)

	0 points	1 point	2 points	points
Patient friendliness	limited	moderate	strong	1
Clinician friendliness	limited	moderate	strong	2
			Subtotal	**3**

Total (out of 10)  **8**

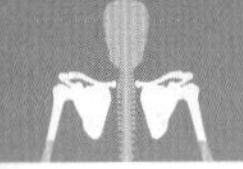

21. Single Assessment Numeric Evaluation (SANE) (1999)

Source: Williams GN, Gangel TJ, Arciero RA, Uhorchak JM, Taylor DC (1999) Comparison of the Single Assessment Numeric Evaluation method and two shoulder rating scales. Outcomes measures after shoulder surgery.
Am J Sports Med; 27:214–221.

Content

Type Patient reported outcome

Single question:
"On a scale of 0 to 100, how would you rate your shoulder function with 100 being normal?"

Interpretation

Minimum score: 0 points
Maximum score: 100 points

The higher the score, the higher the function.

Validation

Outcomes validated against

- ASES
- Rowe shoulder score

Patient population tested in	Validity	Reliability	Responsiveness
Patients who underwent shoulder surgery for instability or significant AC separations (20 years; 90% male)	+	not tested	+

Validation study:
Williams GN, Gangel TJ, Arciero RA, et al (1999) Comparison of the Single Assessment Numeric Evaluation method and two shoulder rating scales. Outcomes measures after shoulder surgery. Am J Sports Med; 27:214–221.

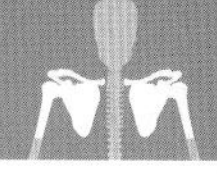

Methodological evaluation ●●○○○○ (2/6)

		no score	0 points	1 point	points
Validity	Content validity	not tested	not valid	valid	-
	Construct validity	not tested	not valid	valid	-
	Criterion validity	not tested	not valid	valid	1
Reliability	Internal consistency	not tested	not consistent	consistent	-
	Reproducibility	not tested	not reproducible	reproducible	-
	Responsiveness	not tested	not responsive	responsive	1
				Subtotal	**2**

Clinical utility ●●●● (4/4)

	0 points	1 point	2 points	points
Patient friendliness	limited	moderate	strong	2
Clinician friendliness	limited	moderate	strong	2
			Subtotal	**4**

Total (out of 10) ●●●●●●○○○○ **6**

22. Subjective Shoulder Rating System (SSRS) (1997)

Source: Kohn D, Geyer M (1997) The subjective shoulder rating system. Arch Orthop Trauma Surg; 116:324–328.

Content

Type Patient reported outcome
Scale 5 subscales (5 items):

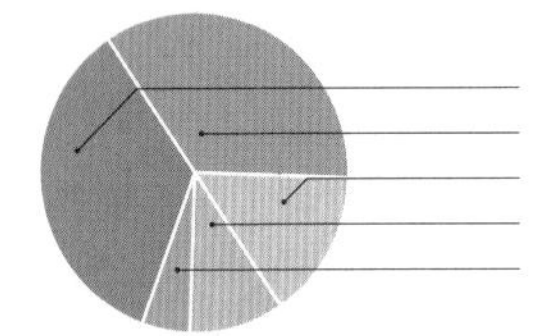

Interpretation

Minimum score: 0 points
Maximum score: 100 points

The higher the score, the higher the function.

Validation

Outcomes validated against

- Constant-Murley shoulder score
- Verbal Rating Score (VRS)

Patient population tested in	Validity	Reliability	Responsiveness
Patients who underwent anterior shoulder reconstructions, subacromial decompression or manipulation under anesthesia (43 years; 59% male)	+	not tested	not tested

Validation study:
Kohn D, Geyer M (1997) The subjective shoulder rating system. Arch Orthop Trauma Surg; 116:324–328.

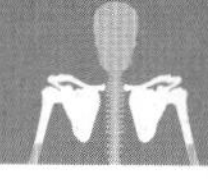

22. Subjective Shoulder Rating System (SSRS) (1997)

Methodological evaluation ●●○○○○ (2/6)

		no score	0 points	1 point	points
Validity	Content validity	**not tested**	not valid	valid	-
	Construct validity	not tested	not valid	**valid**	1
	Criterion validity	not tested	not valid	**valid**	1
Reliability	Internal consistency	**not tested**	not consistent	consistent	-
	Reproducibility	**not tested**	not reproducible	reproducible	-
	Responsiveness	**not tested**	not responsive	responsive	-
				Subtotal	**2**

Clinical utility ●●●● (4/4)

	0 points	1 point	2 points	points
Patient friendliness	limited	moderate	**strong**	2
Clinician friendliness	limited	moderate	**strong**	2
			Subtotal	**4**

Total (out of 10) ●●●●●●○○○○ **6**

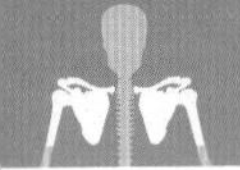

23. Swanson shoulder score (1989)

Source: Swanson AB, de Groot Swanson G, Sattel AB, Cendo RD, Hynes D, Jar-Ning W (1989) Bipolar implant shoulder arthroplasty. Long-term results.
Clin Orthop; 227–247.

Content

Type Clinician based outcome
Scale 3 subscales (8 items):

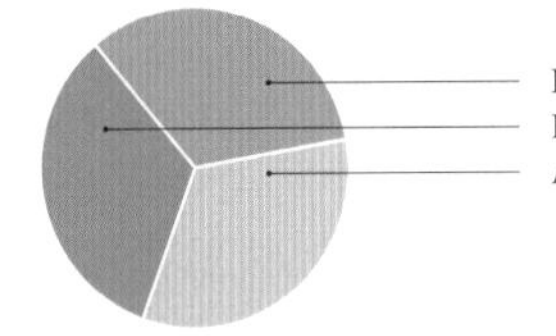

Interpretation

Excellent: 28–30.0 points
Good: 23–27.9 points
Fair: 18–22.9 points
Poor: < 18 points

Validation

No validation studies were identified.

Patient population tested in	Validity	Reliability	Responsiveness
Not applicable			

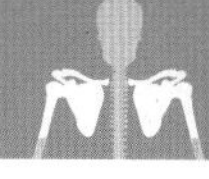

Methodological evaluation

○○○○○○ (0/6)

		no score	0 points	1 point	points
Validity	Content validity	not tested	not valid	valid	-
	Construct validity	not tested	not valid	valid	-
	Criterion validity	not tested	not valid	valid	-
Reliability	Internal consistency	not tested	not consistent	consistent	-
	Reproducibility	not tested	not reproducible	reproducible	-
	Responsiveness	not tested	not responsive	responsive	-
				Subtotal	-

Clinical utility

●●●● (4/4)

	0 points	1 point	2 points	points
Patient friendliness	limited	moderate	strong	2
Clinician friendliness	limited	moderate	strong	2
			Subtotal	4

Total (out of 10) ●●●●○○○○○○ **4**

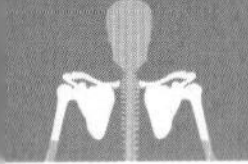

24. UCLA End-Result score (UCLA rating for pain and function of the shoulder) (1986)

Source: Ellman H, Hanker G, Bayer M (1986) Repair of the rotator cuff. End-result study of factors influencing reconstruction. J Bone Joint Surg Am; 68:1136–1144.

Content

Type Clinician based outcome
Scale 5 subscales (5 items):

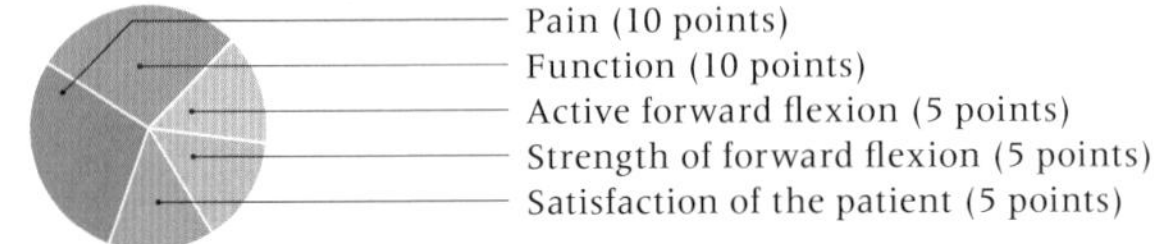

Interpretation

Minimum score: 0 points; maximum score: 35 points
The higher the score, the higher the function.

Validation

Outcomes validated against [1]

- SPADI
- SST

Patient population tested in	Validity	Reliability	Responsiveness
Patients with shoulder disorders (47 years; 58% male) [1]	–	not tested	not tested
Patients with shoulder dysfunction (49.2 years; 65% male) [2]	not tested	+	not tested
Patients who underwent decompression surgery for chronic impingement syndrome (62 years; 46% male) [3]	not tested	not tested	+

Validation studies:

[1] Roddey TS, Olson SL, Cook KF, et al (2000) Comparison of the University of California-Los Angeles Shoulder Scale and the Simple Shoulder Test with the shoulder pain and disability index: single-administration reliability and validity. Phys Ther; 80: 759–768.

[2] Cook KF, Roddey TS, Olson SL, et al (2002) Reliability by surgical status of self-reported outcomes in patients who have shoulder pathologies. J Orthop Sports Phys Ther; 32:336–346.

[3] O'Connor DA, Chipchase LS, Tomlinson J, et al (1999) Arthroscopic subacromial decompression: responsiveness of disease-specific and health-related quality of life outcome measures. Arthroscopy; 15: 836–840.

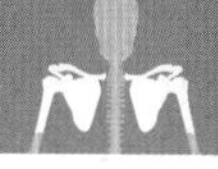

24. UCLA End-Result score (UCLA rating for pain and function of the shoulder) (1986)

Methodological evaluation ●●○○○○ (2/6)

		no score	0 points	1 point	points
Validity	Content validity	**not tested**	not valid	valid	-
	Construct validity	not tested	**not valid**	valid	0
	Criterion validity	**not tested**	not valid	valid	-
Reliability	Internal consistency	**not tested**	not consistent	consistent	-
	Reproducibility	not tested	not reproducible	**reproducible**	1
	Responsiveness	not tested	not responsive	**responsive**	1
				Subtotal	2

Clinical utility ●●●○ (3/4)

	0 points	1 point	2 points	points
Patient friendliness	limited	moderate	**strong**	2
Clinician friendliness	limited	**moderate**	strong	1
			Subtotal	3

Total (out of 10) ●●●●●○○○○○ **5**

25. UCLA shoulder rating score (1981)

Source: Amstutz HC, Sew Hoy AL, Clarke IC (1981) UCLA anatomic total shoulder arthroplasty.
Clin Orthop; (249):227-247.

Content

Type Clinician based outcome
Scale 3 subscales (3 items):

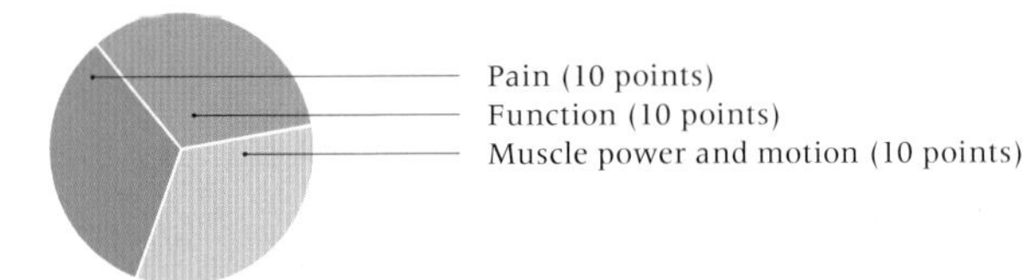

Interpretation

Each subscale graded separately.

Excellent: > 8 points
Good: > 6 points
Fair: > 4 points
Poor: < 3 points

Validation

No validation studies were identified.

Patient population tested in	Validity	Reliability	Responsiveness
Not applicable			

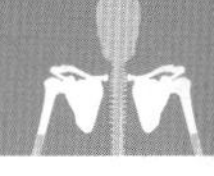

Methodological evaluation ○○○○○○ (0/6)

		no score	0 points	1 point	points
Validity	Content validity	not tested	not valid	valid	-
	Construct validity	not tested	not valid	valid	-
	Criterion validity	not tested	not valid	valid	-
Reliability	Internal consistency	not tested	not consistent	consistent	-
	Reproducibility	not tested	not reproducible	reproducible	-
	Responsiveness	not tested	not responsive	responsive	-
				Subtotal	-

Clinical utility ●●●● (4/4)

	0 points	1 point	2 points	points
Patient friendliness	limited	moderate	strong	2
Clinician friendliness	limited	moderate	strong	2
			Subtotal	**4**

Total (out of 10) ●●●●○○○○○○ **4**

26. Upper extremity function scale (1997)

Source: Pransky G, Feuerstein M, Himmelstein J, Katz JN, Vickers-Lahti M (1997) Measuring functional outcomes in work-related upper extremity disorders. Development and validation of the Upper Extremity Function Scale.
J Occup Environ Med; 39:1195–11202.

Content

Type Patient reported outcome
Scale 8 items:

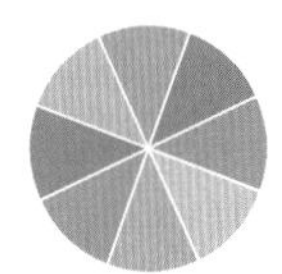

8 items representing common activities affecting upper extremity function (1 to 10 points each).

Interpretation
Minimum score: 8 points
Maximum score: 80 points

The higher the score, the lower the function.

Validation

Outcomes validated against
- Physical findings (grip, pinch, and Phalen's test)
- Duration of symptoms
- Working status
- Arthritis impact measurement scale

Patient population tested in	Validity	Reliability	Responsiveness
Patients with work related upper extremity disorders (38 years; 34% male)	+	+	+
Patients with carpal tunnel syndrome (46 years; 33% male)	+	+	+

Validation study:
Pransky G, Feuerstein M, Himmelstein J, Katz JN, Vickers-Lahti M (1997) Measuring functional outcomes in work-related upper extremity disorders. Development and validation of the Upper Extremity Function Scale.
J Occup Environ Med; 39:1195–1202.

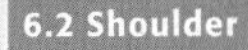

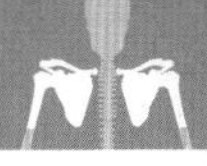

Methodological evaluation ●●●●○○ (4/6)

		no score	0 points	1 point	points
Validity	Content validity	not tested	not valid	**valid**	1
	Construct validity	not tested	not valid	**valid**	1
	Criterion validity	**not tested**	not valid	valid	-
Reliability	Internal consistency	not tested	not consistent	**consistent**	1
	Reproducibility	**not tested**	not reproducible	reproducible	-
	Responsiveness	not tested	not responsive	**responsive**	1
				Subtotal	**4**

Clinical utility ●●●● (4/4)

	0 points	1 point	2 points	points
Patient friendliness	limited	moderate	**strong**	2
Clinician friendliness	limited	moderate	**strong**	2
			Subtotal	**4**

Total (out of 10) ●●●●●●●●○○ **8**

27. Upper extremity functional limitation scale (2001)

Source: Simonsick EM, Kasper JD, Guralnik JM, Bandeen-Roche K, Ferrucci L, Hirsch R, Leveille S, Rantanen T, Fried LP (2001) Severity of upper and lower extremity functional limitation: scale development and validation with self-report and performance-based measures of physical function. WHAS Research Group. Women's Health and Aging Study.
J Gerontol B Psychol Sci Soc Sci; 56:S10–19.

Content

Type Patient reported outcome
Scale 7 items:

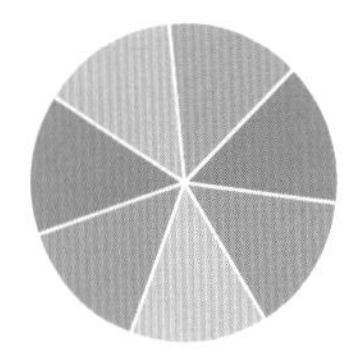

7 items relating to activities of daily living (0 to 4 points each).
Likert scale for each item (4 choices).

Interpretation

Scoring algorithm available upon request from author.

Validation

Outcomes validated against

- Using fingers to grasp or handle
- Lifting and carrying 10 pounds
- Raising arms up over head

Patient population tested in	Validity	Reliability	Responsiveness
Elderly women (≥ 65 yrs) reporting difficulty with mobility and activities of daily living (age NR; 0% male)	+	not tested	not tested

Validation study:

Simonsick EM, Kasper JD, Guralnik JM, et al (2001) Severity of upper and lower extremity functional limitation: scale development and validation with self-report and performance-based measures of physical function. WHAS Research Group. Women's Health and Aging Study. J Gerontol B Psychol Sci Soc Sci; 56:S10–19.

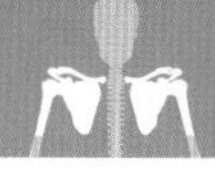

Methodological evaluation ●●○○○○ (2/6)

		no score	0 points	1 point	points
Validity	Content validity	not tested	not valid	**valid**	1
	Construct validity	**not tested**	not valid	valid	-
	Criterion validity	not tested	not valid	**valid**	1
Reliability	Internal consistency	**not tested**	not consistent	consistent	-
	Reproducibility	**not tested**	not reproducible	reproducible	-
	Responsiveness	**not tested**	not responsive	responsive	-
				Subtotal	**2**

Clinical utility ●●●● (4/4)

	0 points	1 point	2 points	points
Patient friendliness	limited	moderate	**strong**	2
Clinician friendliness	limited	moderate	**strong**	2
			Subtotal	**4**

Total (out of 10) ●●●●●●○○○○ **6**

28. Wolfgang criteria for rating results of rotator cuff surgical repair (1974)

Source: Wolfgang GL (1974) Surgical repair of tears of the rotator cuff of the shoulder. Factors influencing the result.
J Bone Joint Surg Am; 56:14–26.

Content

Type Clinician based outcome
Scale 5 subscales (5 items):

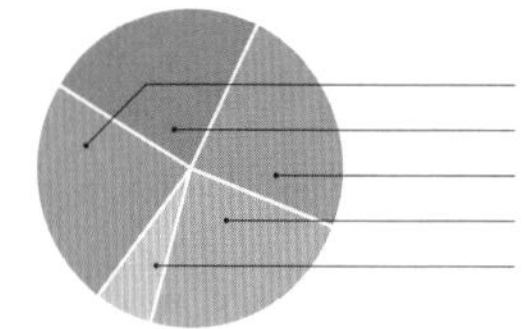

Interpretation
Excellent: 14–17 points
Good: 11–13 points
Fair: 8–10 points
Poor: < 8 points

Validation

No validation studies were identified.

Patient population tested in	Validity	Reliability	Responsiveness
Not applicable			

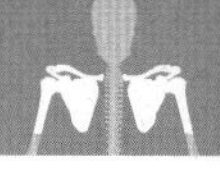

Methodological evaluation ○○○○○○ (0/6)

		no score	0 points	1 point	points
Validity	Content validity	not tested	not valid	valid	-
	Construct validity	not tested	not valid	valid	-
	Criterion validity	not tested	not valid	valid	-
Reliability	Internal consistency	not tested	not consistent	consistent	-
	Reproducibility	not tested	not reproducible	reproducible	-
	Responsiveness	not tested	not responsive	responsive	-
				Subtotal	-

Clinical utility ●●●○ (3/4)

	0 points	1 point	2 points	points
Patient friendliness	limited	moderate	strong	2
Clinician friendliness	limited	moderate	strong	1
			Subtotal	3

Total (out of 10) ●●●○○○○○○○ **3**

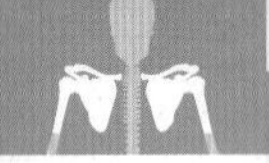

29. Western Ontario Osteoarthritis of the Shoulder index (WOOS) (2001)

Source: Lo IK, Griffin S, Kirkley A (2001) The development of a disease-specific quality of life measurement tool for osteoarthritis of the shoulder: The Western Ontario Osteoarthritis of the Shoulder (WOOS) index.
Osteoarthritis Cartilage; 9:771–778.

Content

Type Patient reported outcome
Scale 4 subscales (19 items):

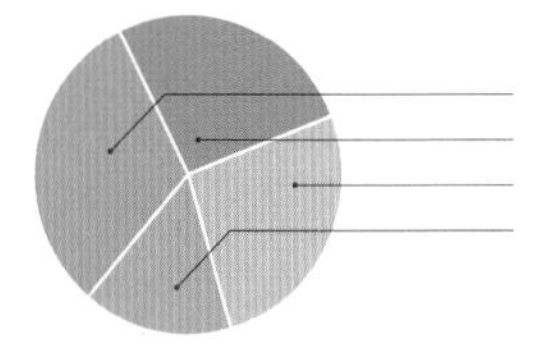

All items rated by using a 100 mm VAS.

Interpretation

Maximum score: 1900 points
Minimum score: 0 points

Scores normalized to 100% and reported as a percentage of normal.
The higher the score, the lower the function.
The higher the normalized score, the higher the function.

Validation

Outcomes validated against

- Constant-Murley shoulder score
- UCLA shoulder rating score
- ASES
- SF-12
- McGill Pain and VAS scales
- Global change rating scale
- Range of motion

Patient population tested in	Validity	Reliability	Responsiveness
Patients receiving treatment for osteoarthritis of the shoulder (age NR; % male NR)	+	+	+

Validation study:

Lo IK, Griffin S, Kirkley A (2001) The development of a disease-specific quality of life measurement tool for osteoarthritis of the shoulder: The Western Ontario Osteoarthritis of the Shoulder (WOOS) index. Osteoarthritis Cartilage; 9:771–778.

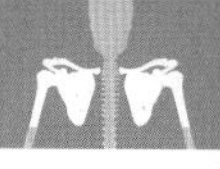

Methodological evaluation ●●●●○○ (4/6)

		no score	0 points	1 point	points
Validity	Content validity	not tested	not valid	valid	1
	Construct validity	not tested	not valid	valid	1
	Criterion validity	not tested	not valid	valid	-
Reliability	Internal consistency	not tested	not consistent	consistent	-
	Reproducibility	not tested	not reproducible	reproducible	1
	Responsiveness	not tested	not responsive	responsive	1
				Subtotal	**4**

Clinical utility ●●●○ (3/4)

	0 points	1 point	2 points	points
Patient friendliness	limited	moderate	strong	1
Clinician friendliness	limited	moderate	strong	2
			Subtotal	**3**

Total (out of 10) 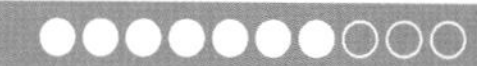 **7**

30. Western Ontario Rotator Cuff (WORC) (2003)

Source: Kirkley A, Alvarez C, Griffin S (2003): The development and evaluation of a disease-specific quality-of-life questionnaire for disorders of the rotator cuff: The Western Ontario Rotator Cuff Index. Clin J Sport Med; 13:84–92.

Content

Type Patient reported outcome
Scale 5 subscales (21 items):

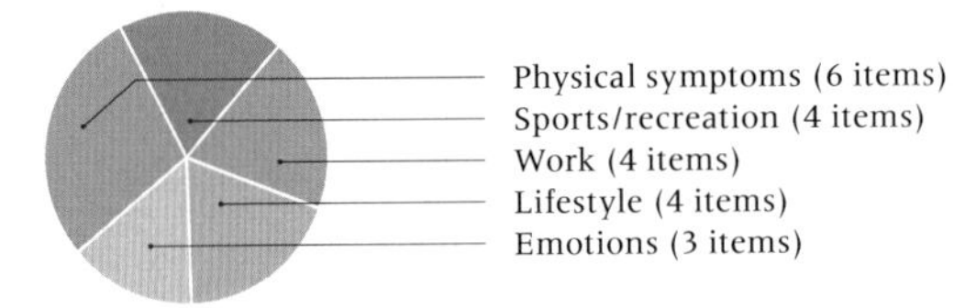

Interpretation

Maximum score: 2100 points
Minimum score: 0 points

Scores normalized to 100% and reported as a percentage of normal.
The higher the score, the lower the function.
The higher the normalized score, the higher the function.

Validation

Outcomes validated against

- SF-36
- UCLA shoulder rating score
- Constant-Murley shoulder score
- ASES
- DASH
- Sickness Impact Profile
- Range of motion

Patient population tested in	Validity	Reliability	Responsiveness
Patients with disability due to disorders of the rotator cuff (age NR; % sex NR)	+	+	+

Validation study:

Kirkley A, Alvarez C, Griffin S (2003): The development and evaluation of a disease-specific quality-of-life questionnaire for disorders of the rotator cuff: The Western Ontario Rotator Cuff Index. Clin J Sport Med; 13:84–92.

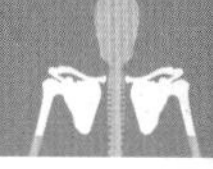

Methodological evaluation

●●●●○○ (4/6)

		no score	0 points	1 point	points
Validity	Content validity	not tested	not valid	**valid**	1
Validity	Construct validity	not tested	not valid	**valid**	1
Validity	Criterion validity	**not tested**	not valid	valid	-
Reliability	Internal consistency	**not tested**	not consistent	consistent	-
Reliability	Reproducibility	not tested	not reproducible	**reproducible**	1
	Responsiveness	not tested	not responsive	**responsive**	1
				Subtotal	**4**

Clinical utility

●●●○ (3/4)

	0 points	1 point	2 points	points
Patient friendliness	limited	moderate	**strong**	2
Clinician friendliness	limited	**moderate**	strong	1
			Subtotal	**3**

Total (out of 10) ●●●●●●●○○○ **7**

31. Western Ontario Instability Index (WOSI) (1998)

Source: Kirkley A, Griffin S, McLintock H, Ng L (1998) The development and evaluation of a disease-specific quality of life measurement tool for shoulder instability. The Western Ontario Shoulder Instability Index (WOSI).
Am J Sports Med; 26:764–772.

Content

Type Patient reported outcome
Scale 4 subscales (21 items)

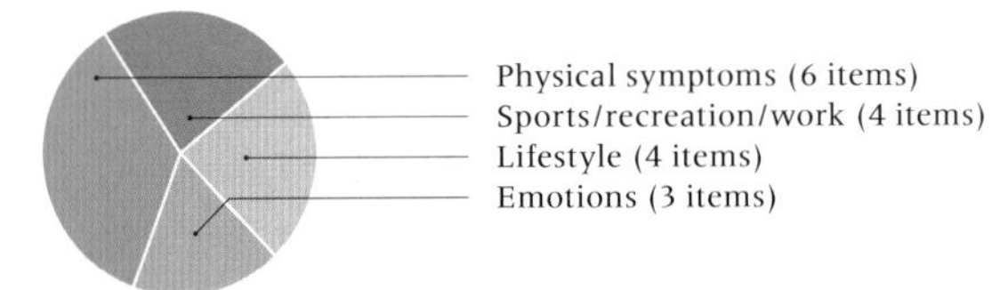

Interpretation

Maximum score: 2100 points
Minimum score: 0 points

Scores normalized to 100% and reported as a percentage of normal.
The higher the score, the lower the function.
The higher the normalized score, the higher the function.

Validation

Outcomes validated against

- DASH
- ASES
- UCLA Shoulder Rating Score
- Rowe Rating Scale
- Constant-Murley shoulder score
- SF-12

Patient population tested in	Validity	Reliability	Responsiveness
Patients who were undergoing treatment for shoulder instability (ae NR; % sex NR)	+	+	+

Validation study:

Kirkley A, Griffin S, McLintock H, et al (1998) The development and evaluation of a disease-specific quality of life measurement tool for shoulder instability. The Western Ontario Shoulder Instability Index (WOSI). Am J Sports Med; 26:764–772.

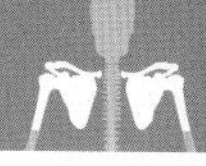

Methodological evaluation ●●●●○○ (4/6)

		no score	0 points	1 point	points
Validity	Content validity	not tested	not valid	**valid**	1
	Construct validity	not tested	not valid	**valid**	1
	Criterion validity	**not tested**	not valid	valid	-
Reliability	Internal consistency	**not tested**	not consistent	consistent	-
	Reproducibility	not tested	not reproducible	**reproducible**	1
	Responsiveness	not tested	not responsive	**responsive**	1
				Subtotal	**4**

Clinical utility ●●●○ (3/4)

	0 points	1 point	2 points	points
Patient friendliness	limited	moderate	**strong**	2
Clinician friendliness	limited	**moderate**	strong	1
			Subtotal	**3**

Total (out of 10) ●●●●●●●○○○ **7**

6.3 Elbow

1. American Shoulder and Elbow Surgeons Elbow Assessment Form (ASES) (1999)

Source: King GJ, Richards RR, Zuckerman JD, Blasier R, Dillman C, Friedman RJ, Gartsman GM, Iannotti JP, Murnahan JP, Mow VC, Woo SL (1999) A standardized method for assessment of elbow function. Research Committee, American Shoulder and Elbow Surgeons. J Shoulder Elbow Surg; 8:351–354.

Content

Type Clinician based outcome
Scale Patient evaluation section; 3 subscales
Physician evaluation section; 4 subscales

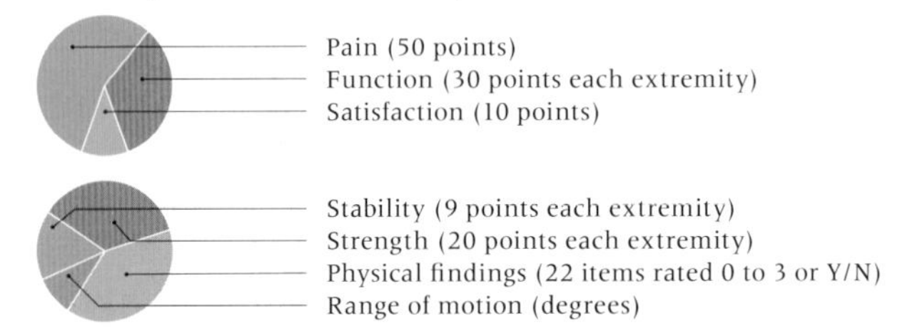

Interpretation
Weighting of subscales or a global score is not reported.

Validation

Outcomes validated against [1]
- Patient rated elbow evaluation
- SF-36
- DASH

Outcomes validated against [2]
- Severity of impairment
- VAS for function and pain
- Mayo clinic performance index for the elbow
- Ewald elbow score
- HSS
- Pritchard scoring system
- Broberg and Morrey elbow scale
- DASH

Patient population tested in	Validity	Reliability	Responsiveness
Patients with elbow disorders (49 years; 47% male) [1]	+	+	not tested
Patients managed operatively and nonoperatively for elbow problems (46 years; 58% male) [2]	+	+	not tested

Validation studies:

[1] MacDermid JC (2001) Outcome evaluation in patients with elbow pathology: issues in instrument development and evaluation. J Hand Ther; 14:105–114.

[2] Turchin DC, Beaton DE, Richards RR (1998) Validity of observer-based aggregate scoring systems as descriptors of elbow pain, function, and disability. J Bone Joint Surg Am; 80:154–162.

1. American Shoulder and Elbow Surgeons Elbow Assessment Form (ASES) (1999)

Methodological evaluation

●●●●○○ (4/6)

		no score	0 points	1 point	points
Validity	Content validity	not tested	not valid	**valid**	1
	Construct validity	not tested	not valid	**valid**	1
	Criterion validity	not tested	not valid	**valid**	1
Reliability	Internal consistency	**not tested**	not consistent	consistent	-
	Reproducibility	not tested	not reproducible	**reproducible**	1
	Responsiveness	**not tested**	not responsive	responsive	-
				Subtotal	**4**

Clinical utility

●●○○ (2/4)

	0 points	1 point	2 points	points
Patient friendliness	limited	moderate	**strong**	2
Clinician friendliness	**limited**	moderate	strong	0
			Subtotal	**2**

Total (out of 10) ●●●●●●○○○○ **6**

2. Bishop rating system (1989)

Source: Kleinman WB, Bishop AT (1989) Anterior intramuscular transposition of the ulnar nerve.
J Hand Srg [Am]; 14:972–979.
Source modified Bishop rating system: Nouhan R, Kleinert JM (1997) Ulnar nerve decompression by transposing the nerve and Z-lengthening the flexor-pronator mass: clinical outcome.
J Hand Surg [Am]; 22(1):127–131.

Content

Type Patient reported outcome
Scale 7 subscales (7 items):

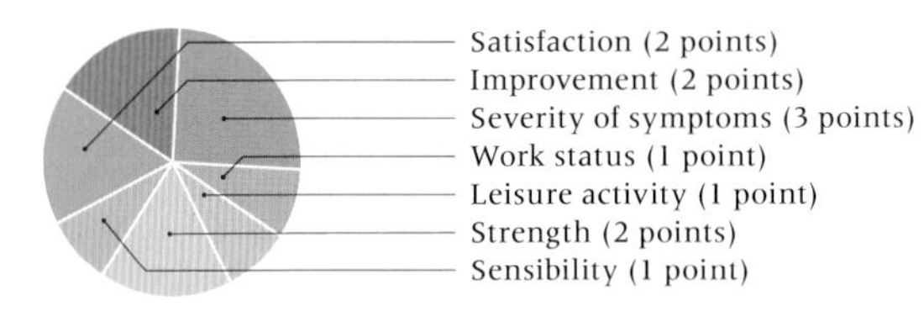

Modified Bishop Scale 5 subscales (5 items):

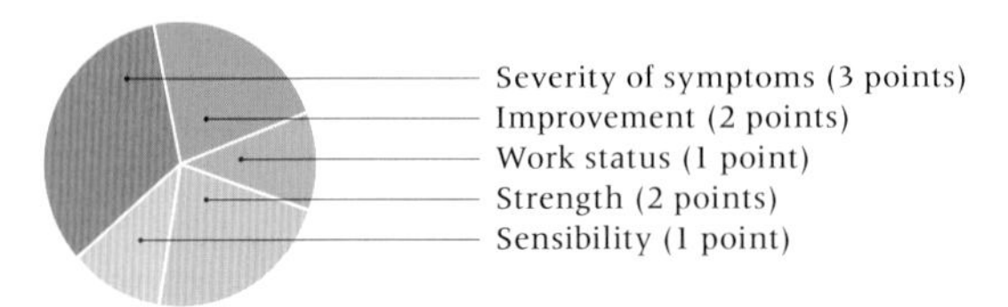

Interpretation

Bishop rating system	Modified Bishop rating system
Excellent: 10–12 points	Excellent: 8–9 points
Good: 7–9 points	Good: 5–7 points
Fair: 4–6 points	Fair: 3–4 points
Poor: 1–3 points	Poor: 0–2

Validation

No validation studies were identified.

Patient population tested in	Validity	Reliability	Responsiveness
Not applicable			

Methodological evaluation ○○○○○○ (0/6)

		no score	0 points	1 point	points
Validity	Content validity	not tested	not valid	valid	-
	Construct validity	not tested	not valid	valid	-
	Criterion validity	not tested	not valid	valid	-
Reliability	Internal consistency	not tested	not consistent	consistent	-
	Reproducibility	not tested	not reproducible	reproducible	-
	Responsiveness	not tested	not responsive	responsive	-
				Subtotal	-

Clinical utility ●●●● (4/4)

	0 points	1 point	2 points	points
Patient friendliness	limited	moderate	strong	2
Clinician friendliness	limited	moderate	strong	2
			Subtotal	**4**

Total (out of 10) ●●●●○○○○○○ **4**

3. Broberg and Morrey elbow scale (1986)

Source: Broberg MA, Morrey BF (1986) Results of delayed excision of the radial head after fracture.
J Bone Joint Surg Am; 68(5):669–674.

Content

Type Clinician based outcome
Scale 4 subscales (4 items):

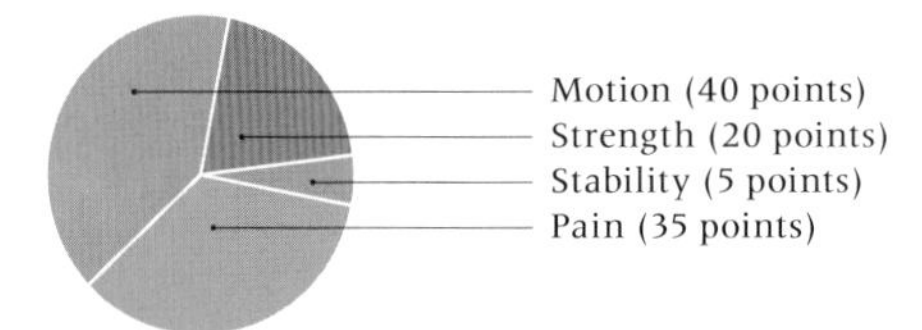

Interpretation
Excellent: 95–100 points
Good: 80–94 points
Fair: 60–79 points
Poor: < 60 points

Validation

Outcomes validated against
- Severity of impairment
- VAS for function and pain
- Ewald elbow score
- HSS
- Pritchard scoring system

Patient population tested in	Validity	Reliability	Responsiveness
Patients managed operatively and nonoperatively for elbow problems (46 years; 58% male)	+/-	not tested	not tested

Validation study:
Turchin DC, Beaton DE, Richards RR (1998) Validity of observer-based aggregate scoring systems as descriptors of elbow pain, function, and disability. J Bone Joint Surg Am; 80:154–162.

Methodological evaluation

●○○○○○ (1/6)

		no score	0 points	1 point	points
Validity	Content validity	**not tested**	not valid	valid	-
	Construct validity	not tested	**not valid**	valid	0
	Criterion validity	not tested	not valid	**valid**	1
Reliability	Internal consistency	**not tested**	not consistent	consistent	-
	Reproducibility	**not tested**	not reproducible	reproducible	-
	Responsiveness	**not tested**	not responsive	responsive	-
				Subtotal	**1**

Clinical utility

●●●○ (3/4)

	0 points	1 point	2 points	points
Patient friendliness	limited	moderate	**strong**	2
Clinician friendliness	limited	**moderate**	strong	1
			Subtotal	**3**

Total (out of 10) 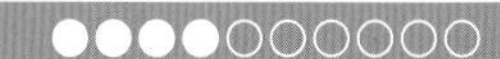 **4**

4. Disabilities of the Arm, Shoulder and Hand (DASH) (1996)

Quick DASH see page 154.

Source: Hudak PL, Amadio PC, Bombardier C (1996) Development of an upper extremity outcome measure: the DASH (disabilities of the arm, shoulder and hand) [corrected]. The Upper Extremity Collaborative Group (UECG).
Am J Ind Med; 29(6):602–608.

Other versions available: Chinese, Dutch, French, German, Hebrew, Italian, Norwegian, Spanish, Swedish, Taiwan Chinese, Turkish.
http://www.dash.iwh.on.ca

Content

Type Patient reported outcome
3 modules (3 required, two optional)

Module 1: ability to perform (required)
Scale 6 subscales (30 items):

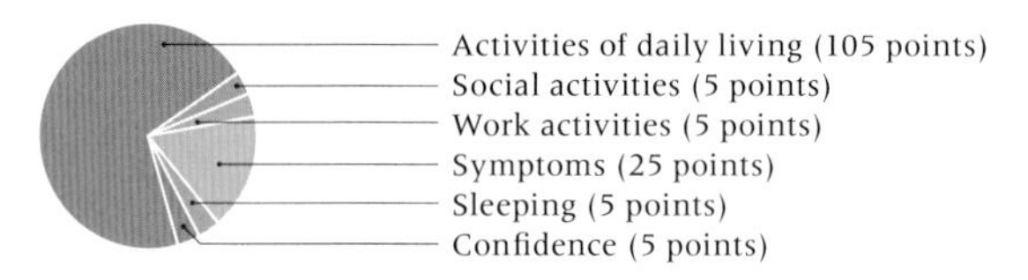

Module 2: ability to perform sports/performing arts (optional)
Scale
Sports/performing arts (20 points)

Module 3: ability to perform work (optional)
Scale
Work (20 points)

Interpretation
Each module is scored separately.

Normalized to 100:
[(Sum of responses / number of completed responses) – 1] × 25 = DASH score

Minimum score: 0 points
Maximum score: 100 points

The higher the score, the lower the function.

Validation

Outcomes validated against [1]
- Severity of impairment
- VAS for function and pain
- Mayo clinic performance index for the elbow
- Ewald elbow score
- HSS
- Pritchard scoring system
- Broberg and Morrey elbow scale
- ASES

Outcomes validated against [2]
- Mayo clinic performance index for the elbow
- SF-36

Outcomes validated against [3]
- ASES
- SF-36
- Patient rated elbow evaluation

Patient population tested in	Validity	Reliability	Responsiveness
Patients managed operatively and nonoperatively for elbow problems (46 years; 58% male) [1]	+	+	not tested
Patients who underwent arthrolysis of the elbow (33 years; 68% male) [2]	+	not tested	not tested
Patients with elbow disorders (49 years; 47% male) [3]	+	not tested	not tested
Patients with upper-extremity conditions planned for surgery (52 years; 42% male) [4]	not tested	+	+

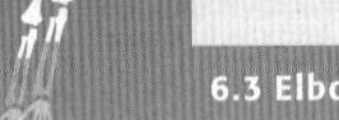

Validation (cont)

Validation studies:

[1] Turchin DC, Beaton DE, Richards RR (1998) Validity of observer-based aggregate scoring systems as descriptors of elbow pain, function, and disability. J Bone Joint Surg Am; 80: 154–162.
[2] Gosling T, Blauth M, Lange T, Richter M, Bastian L, Krettek C (2004) Outcome assessment after arthrolysis of the elbow. Arch Orthop Trauma Surg; 124(4):232–236.
[3] MacDermid JC (2001) Outcome evaluation in patients with elbow pathology: issues in instrument development and evaluation.
[4] Gummesson C, Atroshi I, Ekdahl C (2003) The disabilities of the arm, shoulder and hand (DASH) outcome questionnaire: longitudinal construct validity and measuring self-rated health change after surgery. BMC Musculoskelet Disord; 4(1):11.

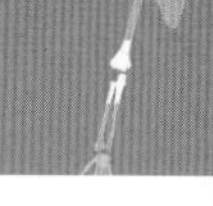

Methodological evaluation ●●●●●○ (5/6)

		no score	0 points	1 point	points
Validity	Content validity	not tested	not valid	valid	1
	Construct validity	not tested	not valid	valid	1
	Criterion validity	not tested	not valid	valid	-
Reliability	Internal consistency	not tested	not consistent	consistent	1
	Reproducibility	not tested	not reproducible	reproducible	1
	Responsiveness	not tested	not responsive	responsive	1
				Subtotal	**5**

Clinical utility ●●○○ (2/4)

	0 points	1 point	2 points	
Patient friendliness	limited	moderate	strong	0
Clinician friendliness	limited	moderate	strong	2
			Subtotal	**2**

Total (out of 10) 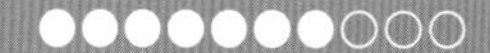 **7**

5. Elbow Functional Assessment scale (EFA) (1999)

Source: de Boer YA, van den Ende CH, Eygendaal D, Jolie IM, Hazes JM, Rozing PM (1999) Clinical reliability and validity of elbow functional assessment in rheumatoid arthritis.
J Rheumatol; 26(9):1909–1917.

Content

Type Clinician based outcome
Scale 3 subscales (12 items):

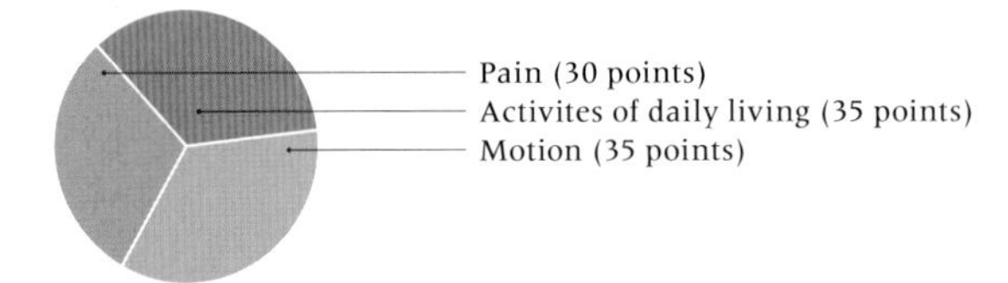

Interpretation
Minimum score: 0 points
Maximum score: 100 points
The higher the score, the higher the function.

Validation

Outcomes validated against [1]

- HSS
- HSS2
- Mayo clinic performance index for the elbow

Patient population tested in	Validity	Reliability	Responsiveness
Rheumatoid arthritis patients with elbow involvement (60 years; 24% male) [1]	+	+	not tested
Rheumatoid arthritis patients undergoing elbow arthroplasty or synovectomy (60 years; 24% male) [2]	not tested	not tested	+

Validation studies:

[1] de Boer YA, van den Ende CH, Eygendaal D, et al (1999) Clinical reliability and validity of elbow functional assessment in rheumatoid arthritis. J Rheumatol; 26(9):1909–1917.
[2] de Boer YA, Hazes JM, Winia PC, et al (2001) Comparative responsiveness of four elbow scoring instruments in patients with rheumatoid arthritis. J Rheumatol; 28(12):2616–2623.

Methodological evaluation

●●●●●○ (5/6)

		no score	0 points	1 point	points
Validity	Content validity	not tested	not valid	valid	1
	Construct validity	not tested	not valid	valid	1
	Criterion validity	not tested	not valid	valid	-
Reliability	Internal consistency	not tested	not consistent	consistent	1
	Reproducibility	not tested	not reproducible	reproducible	1
	Responsiveness	not tested	not responsive	responsive	1
				Subtotal	**5**

Clinical utility

●●●● (4/4)

	0 points	1 point	2 points	points
Patient friendliness	limited	moderate	strong	2
Clinician friendliness	limited	moderate	strong	2
			Subtotal	**4**

Total (out of 10) ●●●●●●●●●○ **9**

6. Ewald elbow score (1975)

Source: Ewald FC (1975) Total elbow replacement. Orthop Clin North Am; 6(3):685–696.

Content

Type Clinician based outcome
Scale 4 subscales (5 items):

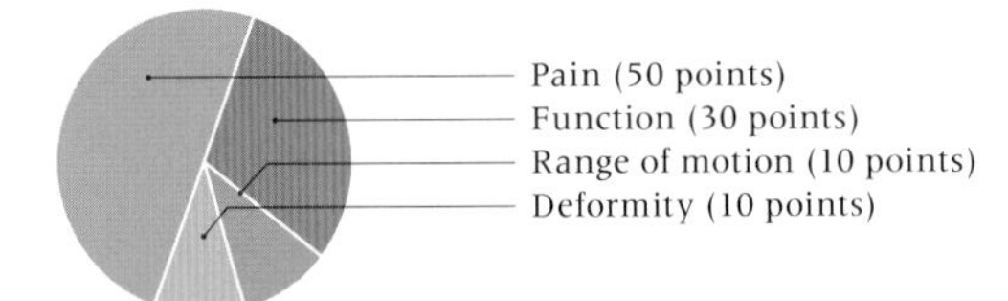

Interpretation

Minimum score: 0 points
Maximum score: 100 points
The higher the score, the higher the function.

Validation

Outcomes validated against

- Severity of impairment
- VAS for function and pain
- Mayo clinic performance index for the elbow
- Broberg and Morrey elbow scale
- HSS
- Pritchard scoring system
- DASH
- ASES

Patient population tested in	Validity	Reliability	Responsiveness
Patients managed operatively and nonoperatively for elbow problems (46 years; 58% male)	+	not tested	not tested

Validation study:
Turchin DC, Beaton DE, Richards RR (1998) Validity of observer-based aggregate scoring systems as descriptors of elbow pain, function, and disability. J Bone Joint Surg Am; 80:154–162.

Methodological evaluation

●●○○○○ (2/6)

		no score	0 points	1 point	points
Validity	Content validity	**not tested**	not valid	valid	-
	Construct validity	not tested	not valid	**valid**	1
	Criterion validity	not tested	not valid	**valid**	1
Reliability	Internal consistency	**not tested**	not consistent	consistent	-
	Reproducibility	**not tested**	not reproducible	reproducible	-
	Responsiveness	**not tested**	not responsive	responsive	-
				Subtotal	2

Clinical utility

●●●○ (3/4)

	0 points	1 point	2 points	points
Patient friendliness	limited	moderate	**strong**	2
Clinician friendliness	limited	**moderate**	strong	1
			Subtotal	3

Total (out of 10) ●●●●●○○○○○ **5**

7. Hospital for Special Surgery assessment scale (HSS) (1980)

Source: Inglis AE, Pellicci PM (1980) Total elbow replacement. J Bone Joint Surg Am; 62(8):1252–1258.

Content

Type Clinician based outcome

Scale 5 subscales (9 items):

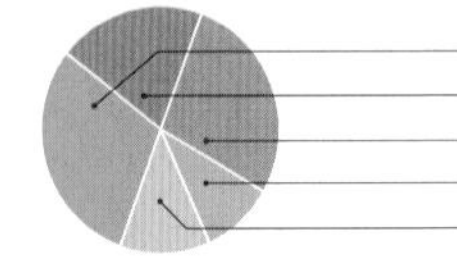

- Pain (30 points)
- Function and activities (20 points)
- Range of motion (28 points)
- Muscle strength (10 points)
- Deformity (12 points)

Interpretation

Minimum score: 0
Maximum score: 100
The higher the score, the higher the function.

Change in score after an intervention can be used to determine effectiveness:

Failure: < 21 point increase
Satisfactory: 21–30 point increase
Good: ≥ 31 point increase

Validation

Outcomes validated against [1]

- Observed elbow function
- Larsen radiological elbow destruction scale

Outcomes validated against [2]

- Severity of impairment
- VAS for function and pain
- Mayo clinic performance index
- Broberg and Morrey scale
- Ewald elbow score
- Pritchard scoring system

Patient population tested in	Validity	Reliability	Responsiveness
Rheumatoid arthritis patients with elbow involvement (60 years; 24% male) [1]	+	+	not tested
Patients managed operatively and nonoperatively for elbow problems (46 years; 58% male) [2]	+/-	not tested	not tested
Rheumatoid arthritis patients with elbow arthroplasty or synovectomy (60 years; 24%male) [3]	not tested	not tested	+

Validation studies:

[1] de Boer YA, van den Ende CH, Eygendaal D, et al (1999) Clinical reliability and validity of elbow functional assessment in rheumatoid arthritis. J Rheumatol; 26(9):1909–1917.

[2] Turchin DC, Beaton DE, Richards RR (1998) Validity of observer-based aggregate scoring systems as descriptors of elbow pain, function, and disability.
J Bone Joint Surg Am; 80:154–162.

[3] de Boer YA, Hazes JM, Winia PC, et al (2001) Comparative responsiveness of four elbow scoring instruments in patients with rheumatoid arthritis. J Rheumatol; 28(12):2616–2623.

7. Hospital for Special Surgery assessment scale (HSS) (1980)

Methodological evaluation

●●●●○○ (4/6)

		no score	0 points	1 point	points
Validity	Content validity	not tested	not valid	valid	-
	Construct validity	not tested	not valid	valid	0
	Criterion validity	not tested	not valid	valid	1
Reliability	Internal consistency	not tested	not consistent	consistent	1
	Reproducibility	not tested	not reproducible	reproducible	1
	Responsiveness	not tested	not responsive	responsive	1
				Subtotal	**4**

Clinical utility

●●●○ (3/4)

	0 points	1 point	2 points	points
Patient friendliness	limited	moderate	strong	2
Clinician friendliness	limited	moderate	strong	1
			Subtotal	**3**

Total (out of 10) ●●●●●●●○○○ **7**

8. Hospital for Special Surgery total elbow scoring system (HSS2) (1990)

Source: Figgie MP, Inglis AE, Mow CS, Wolfe SW, Sculco TP, Figgie HE 3rd (1990)Results of reconstruction for failed total elbow arthroplasty.
Clin Orthop; (253):123–132.

Content

Type Patient reported outcome
Scale 3 subscales (3 items):

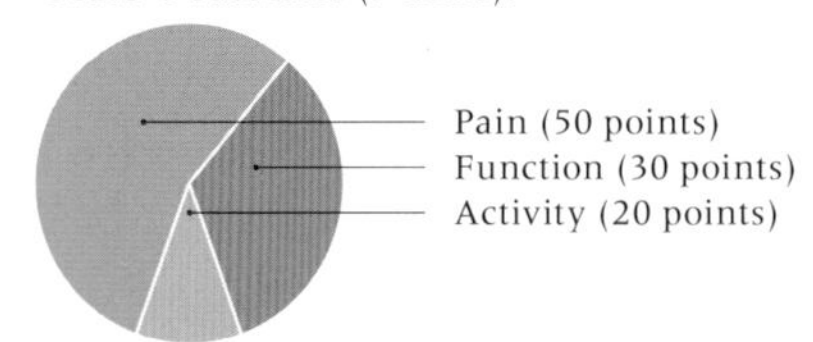

Interpretation
Excellent: 90–100 points
Good: 80–89 points
Fair: 70–79 points
Poor: 60–69 points
Failed: ≤ 59 points

Validation

Outcomes validated against [1]
- Observed elbow function
- Larsen radiological elbow destruction scale

Patient population tested in	Validity	Reliability	Responsiveness
Rheumatoid arthritis patients with elbow involvement (60 years; 24% male) [1]	+	+/-	not tested
Rheumatoid arthritis patients undergoing elbow arthroplasty or synovectomy (60 years; 24%male) [2]	not tested	not tested	+

Validation studies:

[1] de Boer YA, van den Ende CH, Eygendaal D, et al (1999) Clinical reliability and validity of elbow functional assessment in rheumatoid arthritis. J Rheumatol; 26(9):1909–1917.
[2] de Boer YA, Hazes JM, Winia PC, Brand R, Rozing PM (2001) Comparative responsiveness of four elbow scoring instruments in patients with rheumatoid arthritis. J Rheumatol; 28(12):2616–2623.

8. Hospital for Special Surgery total elbow scoring system (HSS2) (1990)

Methodological evaluation

●●●○○○ (3/6)

		no score	0 points	1 point	points
Validity	Content validity	not tested	not valid	valid	-
	Construct validity	not tested	not valid	valid	-
	Criterion validity	not tested	not valid	valid	1
Reliability	Internal consistency	not tested	not consistent	consistent	1
	Reproducibility	not tested	not reproducible	reproducible	0
	Responsiveness	not tested	not responsive	responsive	1
				Subtotal	**3**

Clinical utility

●●●○ (3/4)

	0 points	1 point	2 points	points
Patient friendliness	limited	moderate	strong	2
Clinician friendliness	limited	moderate	strong	1
			Subtotal	**3**

Total (out of 10) ●●●●●●○○○○ **6**

9. Liverpool elbow score (2004)

Source: Sathyamoorthy P, Kemp GJ, Rawal A, Rayner V, Frostick SP (2004) Development and validation of an elbow score. Rheumatology; 43(11):1434–1440.

Content

Type Clinician based outcome
Scale 2 subscales (15 items):

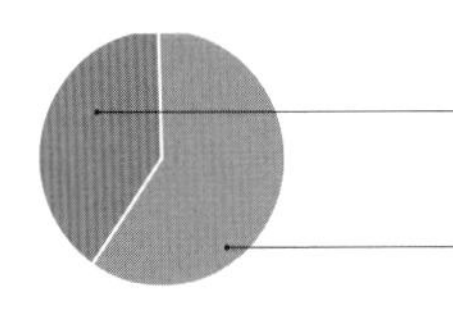

Clinical assessment:
- 6 items evaluating strength, range of motion, and ulna nerve involvement

Patient self-assessment:
- 9 items relating to activities of daily living and pain

Interpretation

All responses are transformed to a scale of 0–10, and equally weighted for summation by averaging.

Minimum score: 0 points
Maximum score: 100 points

Validation

Outcomes validated against

- DASH
- NHP
- SF-12

Patient population tested in	Validity	Reliability	Responsiveness
Patients with various elbow conditions (55 years; 0% male NR)	+	+	+

Validation study:

Sathyamoorthy P, Kemp GJ, Rawal A, et al (2004) Development and validation of an elbow score. Rheumatology; 43(11):1434–1440.

Methodological evaluation

●●●●●○ (5/6)

		no score	0 points	1 point	points
Validity	Content validity	not tested	not valid	valid	1
	Construct validity	not tested	not valid	valid	1
	Criterion validity	not tested	not valid	valid	-
Reliability	Internal consistency	not tested	not consistent	consistent	1
	Reproducibility	not tested	not reproducible	reproducible	1
	Responsiveness	not tested	not responsive	responsive	1
				Subtotal	**5**

Clinical utility

●●●● (4/4)

	0 points	1 point	2 points	points
Patient friendliness	limited	moderate	strong	2
Clinician friendliness	limited	moderate	strong	2
			Subtotal	**4**

Total (out of 10) ●●●●●●●●●○ **9**

10. Mayo clinic performance index for the elbow (1992)

Source: Morrey BF, Adams RA (1992) Semiconstrained arthroplasty for the treatment of rheumatoid arthritis of the elbow. J Bone Joint Surg Am; 74(4):479–490.

Content

Type Clinician based outcome
Scale 4 subscales (8 items):

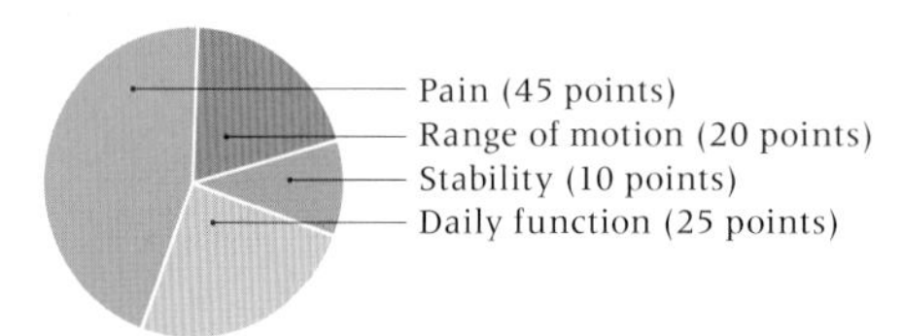

Interpretation

Excellent: 90–100 points
Good: 75–89 points
Fair: 60–74 points
Poor: < 60 points

Validation

Outcomes validated against [1]

- Observed elbow function
- Larsen radiological elbow destruction scale

Outcomes validated against [2]

- Severity of impairment
- VAS for function and pain
- Ewald elbow score
- Broberg and Morrey elbow scale
- HSS
- Pritchard scoring system
- DASH
- ASES

Outcomes validated against [3]

- DASH
- SF-36

Validation (cont)

Patient population tested in	Validity	Reliability	Responsiveness
Rheumatoid arthritis patients with elbow involvement (60 years; 24% male) [1]	-	-	not tested
Patients managed operatively and nonoperatively for elbow problems (46 years; 58% male) [2]	+	not tested	not tested
Patients who underwent arthrolysis of the elbow (33 years; 68%male) [3]	+	not tested	not tested
Rheumatoid arthritis patients undergoing elbow arthroplasty or synovectomy (60 years; 24%male) [4]	not tested	not tested	+

Validation studies:

[1] de Boer YA, van den Ende CH, Eygendaal D, et al (1999) Clinical reliability and validity of elbow functional assessment in rheumatoid arthritis. J Rheumatol; 26(9):1909–1917.

[2] Turchin DC, Beaton DE, Richards RR (1998) Validity of observer-based aggregate scoring systems as descriptors of elbow pain, function, and disability. J Bone Joint Surg Am; 80:154–162.

[3] Gosling T, Blauth M, Lange T, et al (2004) Outcome assessment after arthrolysis of the elbow. Arch Orthop Trauma Surg; 124(4): 232–236.

[4] de Boer YA, Hazes JM, Winia PC, et al (2001) Comparative responsiveness of four elbow scoring instruments in patients with rheumatoid arthritis. J Rheumatol; 28(12):2616–2623.

10. Mayo clinic performance index for the elbow (1992)

Details see previous pages.

Methodological evaluation

●●●○○○ (3/6)

		no score	0 points	1 point	points
Validity	Content validity	**not tested**	not valid	valid	-
	Construct validity	not tested	not valid	**valid**	1
	Criterion validity	not tested	not valid	**valid**	1
Reliability	Internal consistency	not tested	**not consistent**	consistent	0
	Reproducibility	**not tested**	not reproducible	reproducible	-
	Responsiveness	not tested	not responsive	**responsive**	1
				Subtotal	**3**

Clinical utility

●●●○ (3/4)

	0 points	1 point	2 points	points
Patient friendliness	limited	moderate	**strong**	2
Clinician friendliness	limited	**moderate**	strong	1
			Subtotal	**3**

Total (out of 10)  **6**

11. Patient rated elbow evaluation (2001)

Source: MacDermid JC (2001) Outcome evaluation in patients with elbow pathology: issues in instrument development and evaluation. J Hand Ther; 14:105–114.

Content

Type Patient reported outcome
Scale 2 subscales (20 items):

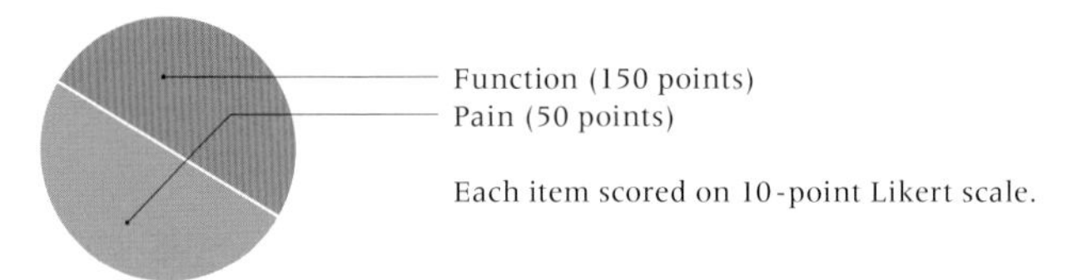

Interpretation

Function subscale normalized to 50 points by dividing by 3.

Minimum score: 0 points
Maximum score: 100 points

The higher the score, the lower the function.

Validation

Outcomes validated against

- ASES
- SF-36
- DASH

Patient population tested in	Validity	Reliability	Responsiveness
Patients with elbow disorders (49 years; 47% male)	+	+	not tested

Validation study:
MacDermid JC (2001) Outcome evaluation in patients with elbow pathology: issues in instrument development and evaluation. J Hand Ther; 14:105–114.

Methodological evaluation

●●●○○○ (3/6)

		no score	0 points	1 point	points
Validity	Content validity	not tested	not valid	valid	1
	Construct validity	not tested	not valid	valid	1
	Criterion validity	not tested	not valid	valid	0
Reliability	Internal consistency	not tested	not consistent	consistent	0
	Reproducibility	not tested	not reproducible	reproducible	1
	Responsiveness	not tested	not responsive	responsive	0
				Subtotal	**3**

Clinical utility

●●●○ (3/4)

	0 points	1 point	2 points	points
Patient friendliness	limited	moderate	strong	1
Clinician friendliness	limited	moderate	strong	2
			Subtotal	**3**

Total (out of 10) ●●●●●●○○○○ **6**

12. Patient rated forearm evaluation (1999)

Source: Overend TJ, Wuori-Fearn JL, Kramer JF, MacDermid JC (1999) Reliability of a patient-rated forearm evaluation questionnaire for patients with lateral epicondylitis.
J Hand Ther; 12(1):31–37.

Content

Type Patient reported outcome
Scale 2 subscales (15 items):

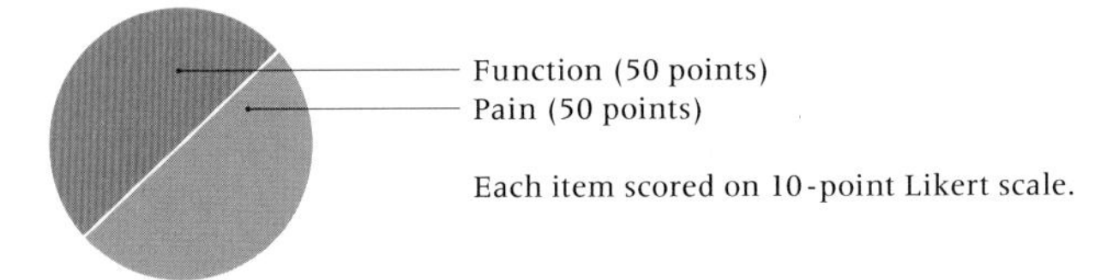

Interpretation

Function subscale normalized to 50 points by dividing by 3.

Minimum score: 0 points
Maximum score: 100 points

The higher the score, the lower the function.

Validation

Outcomes validated against

- Pain-free grip strength

Patient population tested in	Validity	Reliability	Responsiveness
Patients with lateral epicondylitis (45 years; 51% male)	+/-	+	not tested

Validation study:
Overend TJ, Wuori-Fearn JL, Kramer JF, et al (1999) Reliability of a patient-rated forearm evaluation questionnaire for patients with lateral epicondylitis. J Hand Ther; 12(1):31–37.

Methodological evaluation

●●○○○○ (2/6)

		no score	0 points	1 point	points
Validity	Content validity	not tested	not valid	**valid**	1
	Construct validity	**not tested**	not valid	valid	-
	Criterion validity	not tested	**not valid**	valid	0
Reliability	Internal consistency	**not tested**	not consistent	consistent	-
	Reproducibility	not tested	not reproducible	**reproducible**	1
	Responsiveness	**not tested**	not responsive	responsive	-
				Subtotal	**2**

Clinical utility

●●●○ (3/4)

	0 points	1 point	2 points	points
Patient friendliness	limited	**moderate**	strong	1
Clinician friendliness	limited	moderate	**strong**	2
			Subtotal	**3**

Total (out of 10) 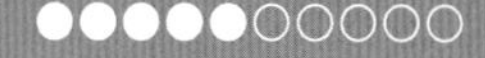 **5**

13. Pritchard scoring system (1977)

Source: Pritchard R (1977) Total Elbow Arthroplasty. In: Joint replacement in the upper extremity.
London: Mechanical engineering publications; p. 67.

Content

Type Clinician based outcome
Scale 3 subscales (5 items):

Range of motion (25 points)
Pain (50 points)
Strength (25 points)

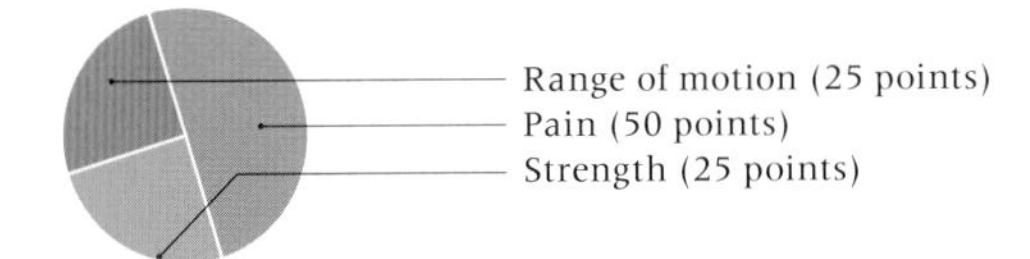

Interpretation

Excellent: 85–100 points
Good: 65–84 points
Poor: < 65 points

Validation

Outcomes validated against

- Severity of impairment
- VAS for function and pain
- Ewald elbow score
- HSS
- DASH
- ASES

Patient population tested in	Validity	Reliability	Responsiveness
Patients managed operatively and nonoperatively for elbow problems (46 years; 58% male)	+/-	not tested	not tested

Validation study:

Turchin DC, Beaton DE, Richards RR (1998) Validity of observer-based aggregate scoring systems as descriptors of elbow pain, function, and disability. J Bone Joint Surg Am; 80:154–162.

Methodological evaluation

●○○○○○ (1/6)

		no score	0 points	1 point	points
Validity	Content validity	not tested	not valid	valid	-
	Construct validity	not tested	not valid	valid	0
	Criterion validity	not tested	not valid	valid	1
Reliability	Internal consistency	not tested	not consistent	consistent	-
	Reproducibility	not tested	not reproducible	reproducible	-
	Responsiveness	not tested	not responsive	responsive	-
				Subtotal	**1**

Clinical utility

●●●● (4/4)

	0 points	1 point	2 points	points
Patient friendliness	limited	moderate	strong	2
Clinician friendliness	limited	moderate	strong	2
			Subtotal	**4**

Total (out of 10) ●●●●●○○○○○ **5**

14. Quick DASH (1996)

Source: King GJ, Richards RR, Zuckerman JD, Blasier R, Dillman C, Friedman RJ, Gartsman GM, Iannotti JP, Murnahan JP, Mow VC, Woo SL (1999) A standardized method for assessment of elbow function. Research Committee, American Shoulder and Elbow Surgeons. J Shoulder Elbow Surg; 8:351–354.

Content

3 modules
Module 1: ability to perform (required)
Scale 5 subscales (11 items):

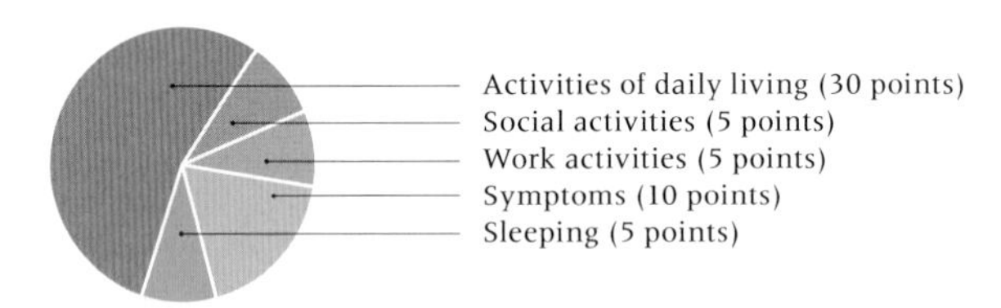

Module 2: ability to perform sports/performing arts (optional)
Scale
Sports/performing arts (20 points)

Module 3: ability to perform work (optional)
Scale
Work (20 points)

Interpretation
Each module is scored separately

Normalized to 100:
[(Sum of responses / number of completed responses) – 1] X 25 = Quick DASH score

Minimum score: 0 points
Maximum score: 100 points

The higher the score, the lower the function.

Validation

No validation studies were identified.

Methodological evaluation

○○○○○○ (0/6)

		no score	0 points	1 point	points
Validity	Content validity	not tested	not valid	valid	-
	Construct validity	not tested	not valid	valid	-
	Criterion validity	not tested	not valid	valid	-
Reliability	Internal consistency	not tested	not consistent	consistent	-
	Reproducibility	not tested	not reproducible	reproducible	-
	Responsiveness	not tested	not responsive	responsive	-
				Subtotal	-

Clinical utility

●●●○ (3/4)

	0 points	1 point	2 points	points
Patient friendliness	limited	moderate	strong	1
Clinician friendliness	limited	moderate	strong	2
			Subtotal	3

Total (out of 10) 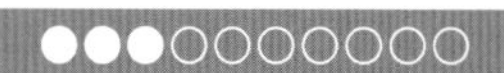 **3**

15. Upper extremity function scale (1997)

Source: Pransky G, Feuerstein M, Himmelstein J, Katz JN, Vickers-Lahti M (1997) Measuring functional outcomes in work-related upper extremity disorders. Development and validation of the Upper Extremity Function Scale.
J Occup Environ Med; 39:1195–11202.

Content

Type Patient reported outcome
Scale 8 items:

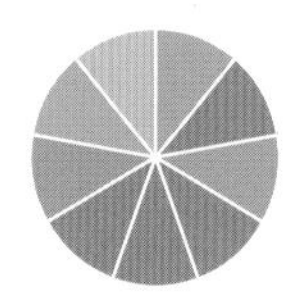

8 items representing common activities affecting upper extremity function (1 to 10 points each).

Interpretation

Minimum score: 8 points
Maximum score: 80 points

The higher the score, the lower the function.

Validation

Outcomes validated against

- Physical findings (grip, pinch, and Phalen's test)
- Duration of symptoms
- Working status
- Arthritis impact measurement scale

Patient population tested in	Validity	Reliability	Responsiveness
Patients with work related upper extremity disorders (38 years; 34% male)	+	+	+
Patients with carpal tunnel syndrome (46 years; 33% male)	+	+	+

Validation study:

Pransky G, Feuerstein M, Himmelstein J, Katz JN, Vickers-Lahti M (1997) Measuring functional outcomes in work-related upper extremity disorders. Development and validation of the Upper Extremity Function Scale.
J Occup Environ Med; 39:1195–1202.

Methodological evaluation

●●●●○○ (4/6)

		no score	0 points	1 point	points
Validity	Content validity	not tested	not valid	valid	1
	Construct validity	not tested	not valid	valid	1
	Criterion validity	not tested	not valid	valid	-
Reliability	Internal consistency	not tested	not consistent	consistent	1
	Reproducibility	not tested	not reproducible	reproducible	-
	Responsiveness	not tested	not responsive	responsive	1
				Subtotal	**4**

Clinical utility

●●●● (4/4)

	0 points	1 point	2 points	points
Patient friendliness	limited	moderate	strong	2
Clinician friendliness	limited	moderate	strong	2
			Subtotal	**4**

Total (out of 10)  **8**

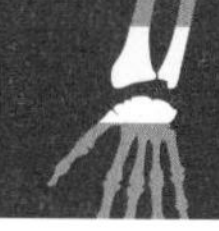

6.4 Wrist/hand

1. Arab hand function index (2004)

Source: Guermazi M, Kessomtini W, Poiraudeau S, Elleuch M, Fermarian J, Elleuch MH, Revel M (2004) Development and validation of an Arabic rheumatoid hand disability scale.
Disabil Rehabil; 26:655–661.

Content

Type Patient reported outcome
Scale 1 subscale (10 items):

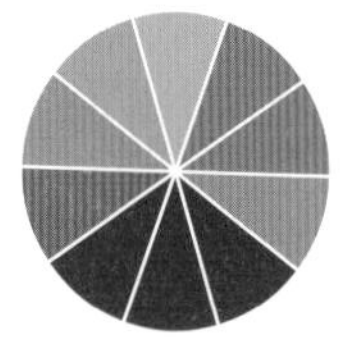

10 questions relating to hand function and activities of daily living.

Likert scale for each item
(4 choices; 0 to 3 points each).

Interpretation

Minimum score: 0 points
Maximum score: 30 points

The higher the score, the lower the function.

Validation

Outcomes validated against

- Revel's function index
- Lee's functional index

Patient population tested in	Validity	Reliability	Responsiveness
Patients with rheumatoid arthritis for at least one year (47.5 years; 13.7% male)	+	+	not tested

Validation study:

Guermazi M, Kessomtini W, Poiraudeau S,et al (2004) Development and validation of an Arabic rheumatoid hand disability scale. Disabil Rehabil; 26:655–661.

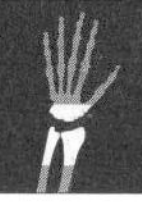

Methodological evaluation

●●●●○○ (4/6)

		no score	0 points	1 point	points
Validity	Content validity	not tested	not valid	**valid**	1
	Construct validity	not tested	not valid	**valid**	1
	Criterion validity	**not tested**	not valid	valid	-
Reliability	Internal consistency	not tested	not consistent	**consistent**	1
	Reproducibility	not tested	not reproducible	**reproducible**	1
	Responsiveness	**not tested**	not responsive	responsive	-
				Subtotal	**4**

Clinical utility

●●●○ (3/4)

	0 points	1 point	2 points	points
Patient friendliness	limited	moderate	**strong**	2
Clinician friendliness	limited	**moderate**	strong	1
			Subtotal	**3**

Total (out of 10) 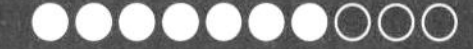 **7**

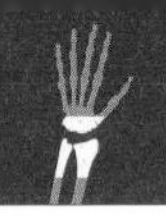

2. Boston questionnaire (also known as Brigham and Women's carpal tunnel questionnaire) (1993)

Source: Levine DW, Simmons BP, Koris MJ, Daltroy LH, Hohl GG, Fossel AH, Katz JN (1993) A self-administered questionnaire for the assessment of severity of symptoms and functional status in carpal tunnel syndrome.
J Bone Joint Surg Am; 75:1585–1592

Other versions available: Swedish.

Content

Type Patient reported outcome
Scale 2 subscales (19 items):

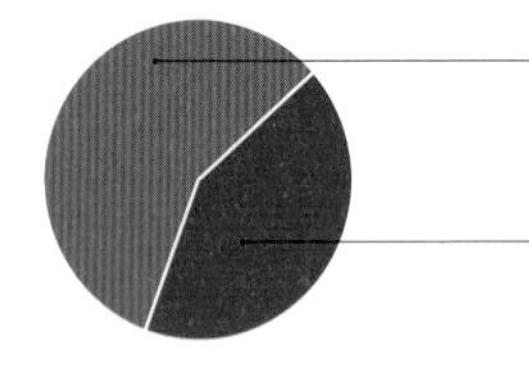

11 symptom severity items pertaining to:
- Pain
- Numbness
- Weakness

8 functional status items pertaining to common activites of daily living.
Each item scored on 1 to 5-point Likert scale.

Interpretation

Each subscale scored separately.
Subscale overall score = mean score of all items answered.
The higher the score, the lower the function.

Validation

Outcomes validated against [1]
- Grip strength
- Pinch strength
- Two-point discrimination
- Semmes-Weinstein monofilament testing

Outcomes validated against [2,3]
- SF-36

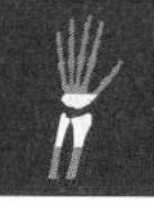

Patient population tested in	Validity	Reliability	Responsiveness
Patients with carpal tunnel syndrome (57 years; 25% male) [1]	+	+	+
Swedish speaking patients undergoing carpal tunnel release (52 years; 34% male) [2]	+	+	+
Patients undergoing surgical treatment for carpal tunnel syndrome (51 years; 26% male) [3]	not tested	not tested	+
Patients undergoing carpal tunnel decompression (58 years; 28% male) [4]	not tested	+	+
Patients undergoing carpal tunnel release (55 years; 45% male) [5]	not tested	not tested	+
Patients scheduled for carpal tunnel release (60 years; 41% male) [6]	not tested	not tested	+

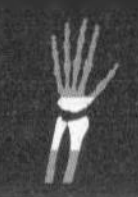

Validation (cont)

Validation studies:

[1] Levine DW, Simmons BP, Koris MJ, et al (1993) A self-administered questionnaire for the assessment of severity of symptoms and functional status in carpal tunnel syndrome. J Bone Joint Surg Am; 75: 1585–1592.
[2] Atroshi I, Johnsson R, Sprinchorn A (1998) Self-administered outcome instrument in carpal tunnel syndrome. Reliability, validity and responsiveness evaluated in 102 patients. Acta Orthop Scand; 69: 82–88.
[3] Atroshi I, Gummesson C, Johnsson R, et al (1999) Symptoms, disability, and quality of life in patients with carpal tunnel syndrome. J Hand Surg [Am], 24: 398–404.
[4] Greenslade JR, Mehta RL, Belward P, et al (2004) Dash and Boston questionnaire assessment of carpal tunnel syndrome outcome: what is the responsiveness of an outcome questionnaire? J Hand Surg [Br]; 29: 159–164.
[5] Gay RE, Amadio PC, Johnson JC (2003) Comparative responsiveness of the disabilities of the arm, shoulder, and hand, the carpal tunnel questionnaire, and the SF-36 to clinical change after carpal tunnel release. J Hand Surg [Am]; 28:250–254.
[6] Amadio PC, Silverstein MD, Ilstrup DM, et al (1996) Outcome assessment for carpal tunnel surgery: the relative responsiveness of generic, arthritis-specific, disease-specific, and physical examination measures. J Hand Surg [Am]; 21: 338–346.

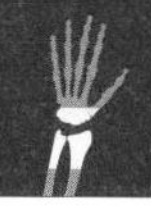

Methodological evaluation

●●●●●○ (5/6)

		no score	0 points	1 point	points
Validity	Content validity	not tested	not valid	**valid**	1
	Construct validity	not tested	not valid	**valid**	1
	Criterion validity	**not tested**	not valid	valid	-
Reliability	Internal consistency	not tested	not consistent	**consistent**	1
	Reproducibility	not tested	not reproducible	**reproducible**	1
	Responsiveness	not tested	not responsive	**responsive**	1
				Subtotal	**5**

Clinical utility

●●●○ (3/4)

	0 points	1 point	2 points	points
Patient friendliness	limited	**moderate**	strong	1
Clinician friendliness	limited	moderate	**strong**	2
			Subtotal	**3**

Total (out of 10) 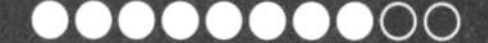 **8**

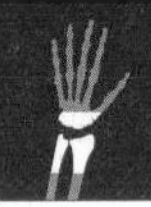

3. Buck-Gramcko/Lohman evaluation for total wrist function (1985)

Source: Buck-Gramcko D, Lohmann H (1985) Compression arthrodesis of the wrist. In: The Hand. Edited by R. Tubiana. Philadelphia: W.B. Saunders Company, pp 723–729.

Content

Type Clinician based outcome
Scale 5 subscales (5 items):

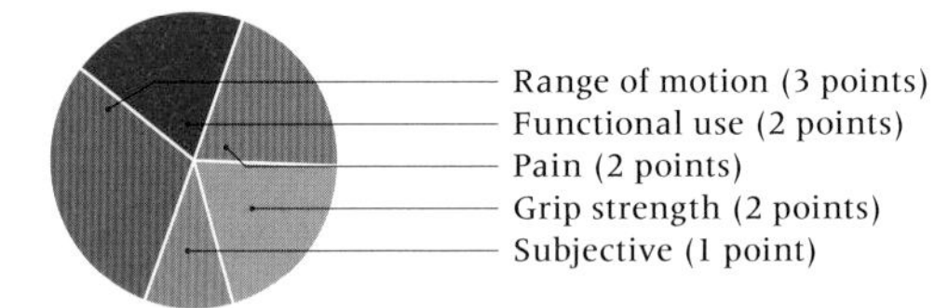

Interpretation
Excellent: 9–10 points
Good: 7–8 points
Satisfactory: 5–6 points
Poor: < 5 points

Validation

No validation studies were identified.

Patient population tested in	Validity	Reliability	Responsiveness
Not applicable			

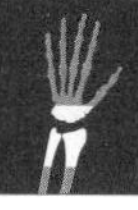

3. Buck-Gramcko/Lohman evaluation for total wrist function (1985)

Methodological evaluation

○○○○○○ (0/6)

		no score	0 points	1 point	points
Validity	Content validity	not tested	not valid	valid	-
	Construct validity	not tested	not valid	valid	-
	Criterion validity	not tested	not valid	valid	-
Reliability	Internal consistency	not tested	not consistent	consistent	-
	Reproducibility	not tested	not reproducible	reproducible	-
	Responsiveness	not tested	not responsive	responsive	-
				Subtotal	-

Clinical utility

●●●○ (3/4)

	0 points	1 point	2 points	points
Patient friendliness	limited	moderate	strong	2
Clinician friendliness	limited	moderate	strong	1
			Subtotal	3

Total (out of 10) 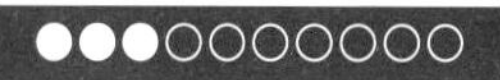 **3**

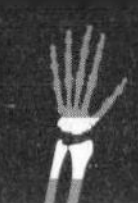

4. Clawson functional index (1971)

Source: Clawson DK, Souter WA, Carthum CJ, Hymen ML (1971)
Functional assessment of the rheumatoid hand.
Clin Orthop; 77:203–210.

Content

Type Clinician based outcome
Scale 5 functional tests (5 items):

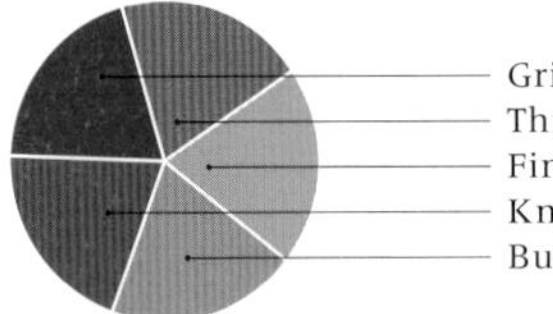

Nondominant hand is subject to all the tests except the Button test.

Interpretation
Each hand scored separately
Nondominant hand score multiplied by 5/4.

Minimum score: 0 points
Maximum score: 100 points

The higher the score, the higher the function.

Validation

No validation studies were identified.

Patient population tested in	Validity	Reliability	Responsiveness
Patients with rheumatoid arthritis (age NR; % male NR)	not tested	not tested	+

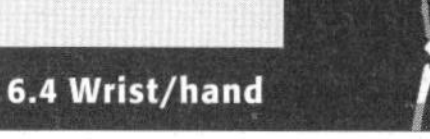

Methodological evaluation

●○○○○○ (1/6)

		no score	0 points	1 point	points
Validity	Content validity	not tested	not valid	valid	-
	Construct validity	not tested	not valid	valid	-
	Criterion validity	not tested	not valid	valid	-
Reliability	Internal consistency	not tested	not consistent	consistent	-
	Reproducibility	not tested	not reproducible	reproducible	-
	Responsiveness	not tested	not responsive	responsive	1
				Subtotal	**1**

Clinical utility

●●●○ (3/4)

	0 points	1 point	2 points	points
Patient friendliness	limited	moderate	strong	2
Clinician friendliness	limited	moderate	strong	1
			Subtotal	**3**

Total (out of 10) 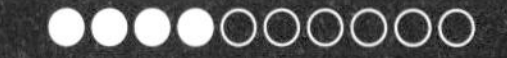 **4**

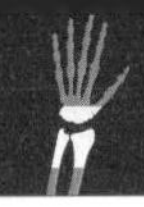

5. Cochin rheumatoid hand disability scale (1996)

Source: Duruoz MT, Poiraudeau S, Fermanian J, Menkes CJ, Amor B, Dougados M, Revel M (1996) Development and validation of a rheumatoid hand functional disability scale that assesses functional handicap.
J Rheumatol; 23:1167–1172.

Other versions available: French.

Content

Type Patient reported outcome
Scale 18 items

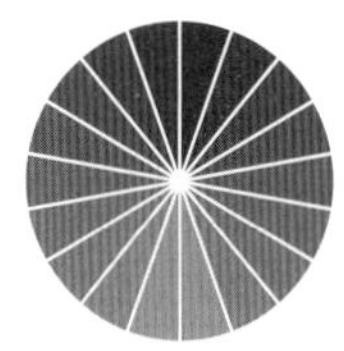

18 items assessing hand function in the following areas:

- In the kitchen
- Dressing
- Hygiene
- In the office
- Other

0 to 5-point Likert scale for each item.

Interpretation

Minimum score: 0 points
Maximum score: 90 points

The higher the score, the lower the function.

Validation

Outcomes validated against [1]

- VAS for functional handicap
- Hand function index

Outcomes validated against [2]

- Kapandji index

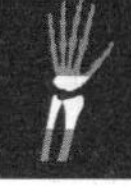

Patient population tested in	Validity	Reliability	Responsiveness
Patients with rheumatoid arthritis (51 years; 18% male) [1]	+	+	not tested
Patients with rheumatoid arthritis of the hand scheduled for surgery (54 years; 16% male) [2]	+	not tested	not tested
Patients with rheumatoid arthritis of the hand scheduled for surgery (54 years; 16% male) [3]	not tested	not tested	+

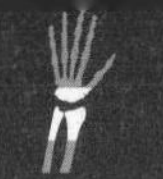

Validation (cont)

Validation studies:

[1] Duruoz MT, Poiraudeau S, Fermanian J, et al (1996) Development and validation of a rheumatoid hand functional disability scale that assesses functional handicap. J Rheumatol; 23:1167–1172.

[2] Lefevre-Colau MM, Poiraudeau S, Oberlin C, et al (2003) Reliability, validity, and responsiveness of the modified Kapandji index for assessment of functional mobility of the rheumatoid hand. Arch Phys Med Rehabil; 84:1032–1038.

[3] Lefevre-Colau MM, Poiraudeau S, Fermanian J, et al (2001) Responsiveness of the Cochin rheumatoid hand disability scale after surgery. Rheumatology (Oxford); 40:843–850.

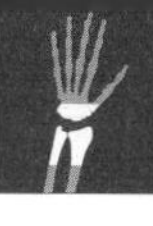

Methodological evaluation

 (5/6)

		no score	0 points	1 point	points
Validity	Content validity	not tested	not valid	valid	1
	Construct validity	not tested	not valid	valid	1
	Criterion validity	not tested	not valid	valid	1
Reliability	Internal consistency	not tested	not consistent	consistent	-
	Reproducibility	not tested	not reproducible	reproducible	1
	Responsiveness	not tested	not responsive	responsive	1
				Subtotal	**5**

Clinical utility

 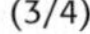 (3/4)

	0 points	1 point	2 points	points
Patient friendliness	limited	moderate	strong	1
Clinician friendliness	limited	moderate	strong	2
			Subtotal	**3**

Total (out of 10) 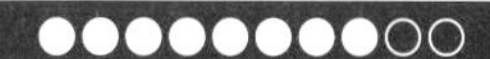 **8**

6. Disabilities of the Arm, Shoulder and Hand (DASH) (1996)

Quick DASH see page 210.

Source: Hudak PL, Amadio PC, Bombardier C (1996) Development of an upper extremity outcome measure: the DASH (disabilities of the arm, shoulder and hand) [corrected]. The Upper Extremity Collaborative Group (UECG).
Am J Ind Med; 29(6):602–608.

Other versions available: Chinese, Dutch, French, German, Hebrew, Italian, Norwegian, Spanish, Swedish, Taiwan Chinese, Turkish.
http://www.dash.iwh.on.ca

Content

Type Patient reported outcome
3 modules (one required, two optional)

Module 1: ability to perform (required)
Scale 6 subscales (30 items):

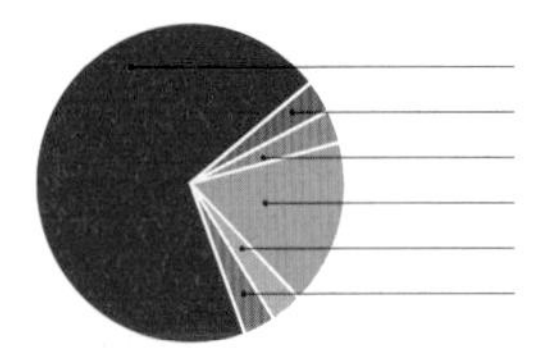

Activities of daily living (105 points)
Social activities (5 points)
Work activities (5 points)
Symptoms (25 points)
Sleeping (5 points)
Confidence (5 points)

Module 2: ability to perform sports/performing arts (optional)
Scale
Sports/performing arts (20 points)

Module 3: ability to perform work (optional)
Scale
Work (20 points)

Interpretation
Each module is scored separately.

Normalized to 100:
[(Sum of responses / number of completed responses) - 1] × 25 = DASH score

Minimum score: 0 points
Maximum score: 100 points

The higher the score, the lower the function.

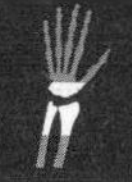

Validation

Outcomes validated against [1]

- Brigham and Women's carpal tunnel questionnaire
- SF-36

Outcomes validated against [2]

- SPADI
- Brigham and Women's carpal tunnel questionnaire
- VAS of pain, function, and ability to work

Patient population tested in	Validity	Reliability	Responsiveness
Patients with surgically managed ulno-carpal impingement in the late post-operative period (34.6 years; 63% male) [1]	+	not tested	not tested
Patients with wrist/hand or shoulder problems (53.6 years; 43% male) [2]	+	+	+
Patients with distal radius fractures (53 years; 37% male) [3]	not tested	not tested	+
Patients scheduled for carpal tunnel release (55 years; 45% male) [4]	not tested	not tested	+
Patients undergoing carpal tunnel decompression (58 years; 28% male) [5]	not tested	+	+

Validation (cont)

Validation studies:

[1] Jain R, Hudak PL, Bowen C, et al (2001) Validity of health status measures in patients with ulnar wrist disorders. J Hand Ther; 14: 147–153.

[2] Greenslade JR, Mehta RL, Belward P, et al (2004) Dash and Boston questionnaire assessment of carpal tunnel syndrome outcome: what is the responsiveness of an outcome questionnaire? J Hand Surg [Br]; 29: 159–164.

[3] MacDermid JC, Richards RS, Donner A, et al (2000) Responsiveness of the short form-36, disability of the arm, shoulder, and hand questionnaire, patient-rated wrist evaluation, and physical impairment measurements in evaluating recovery after a distal radius fracture. J Hand Surg [Am]; 25:330–340.

[4] Gay RE, Amadio PC, Johnson JC (2003) Comparative responsiveness of the disabilities of the arm, shoulder, and hand, the carpal tunnel questionnaire, and the SF-36 to clinical change after carpal tunnel release. J Hand Surg [Am]; 28:250–254.

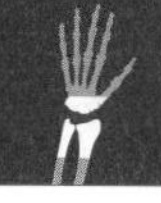

Methodological evaluation

 (5/6)

		no score	0 points	1 point	points
Validity	Content validity	not tested	not valid	**valid**	1
	Construct validity	not tested	not valid	**valid**	1
	Criterion validity	**not tested**	not valid	valid	-
Reliability	Internal consistency	not tested	not consistent	**consistent**	1
	Reproducibility	not tested	not reproducible	**reproducible**	1
	Responsiveness	not tested	not responsive	**responsive**	1
				Subtotal	**5**

Clinical utility

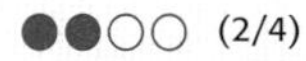 (2/4)

	0 points	1 point	2 points	points
Patient friendliness	**limited**	moderate	strong	0
Clinician friendliness	limited	moderate	**strong**	2
			Subtotal	**2**

Total (out of 10) 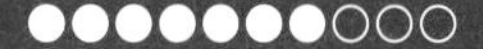 **7**

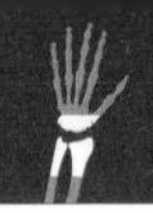

7. Forearm symptom severity scale (1998)

Source: Flinkkila T, Raatikainen T, Hamalainen M (1998) AO and Frykman's classifications of Colles' fracture. No prognostic value in 652 patients evaluated after 5 years.
Acta Orthop Scand; 69:77–81.

Content

Type Patient reported outcome
Scale 9 questions relating to:

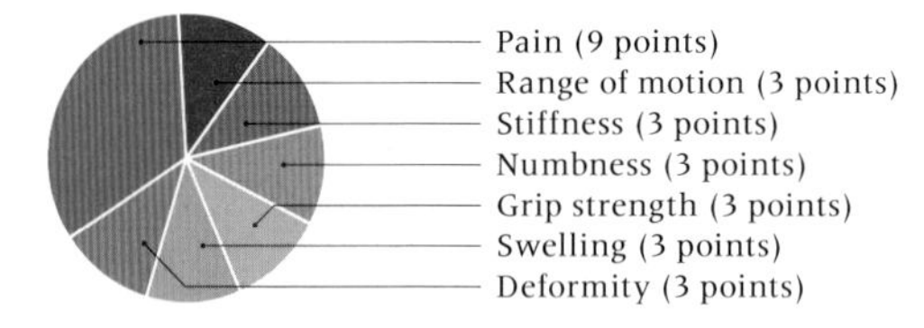

Interpretation

Symptom severity:
None: 0 points
Mild: 1–6 points
Moderate: 7–12 points
Severe: 13–18 points
Very severe: 19–27 points

Validation

No validation studies were identified.

Patient population tested in	Validity	Reliability	Responsiveness
Not applicable			

Methodological evaluation

○○○○○○ (0/6)

		no score	0 points	1 point	points
Validity	Content validity	not tested	not valid	valid	-
	Construct validity	not tested	not valid	valid	-
	Criterion validity	not tested	not valid	valid	-
Reliability	Internal consistency	not tested	not consistent	consistent	-
	Reproducibility	not tested	not reproducible	reproducible	-
	Responsiveness	not tested	not responsive	responsive	-
				Subtotal	-

Clinical utility

●●●● (4/4)

	0 points	1 point	2 points	points
Patient friendliness	limited	moderate	strong	2
Clinician friendliness	limited	moderate	strong	2
			Subtotal	4

Total (out of 10)

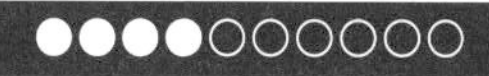

4

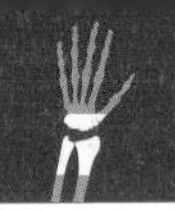

8. Functional index (1951)

Source: Porter ML, Stockley I (1951) Functional index: a numerical expression of post-traumatic wrist function.
Injury; 16:188–192.

Content

Type Clinician based outcome
Scale 3 subscales (3 items):

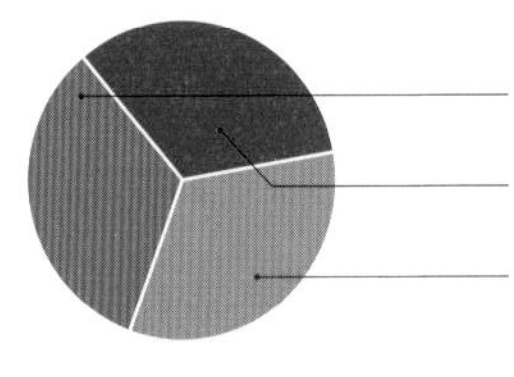

Torque index = dynamometer used for supination/pronation strength (% normal)
Grip index = vigorometer used for grip strength (% normal)
Range of motion index = goniometer used for total range of motion (% normal)

Interpretation

Functional index = (torque index + grip index + range of motion index) / 3

Validation

Outcomes validated against

- Gartland and Werley scoring system
- Patient's subjective categorization of return to function
- Author's subjective categorization of return to function

Patient population tested in	Validity	Reliability	Responsiveness
Patients with fractures of the distal radius (60 years; 20% male)	+	not tested	not tested

Validation study:

Porter ML, Stockley I (1951) Functional index: a numerical expression of post-traumatic wrist function. Injury; 16:188–192.

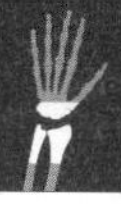

Methodological evaluation ●○○○○○ (1/6)

		no score	0 points	1 point	points
Validity	Content validity	not tested	not valid	valid	-
	Construct validity	not tested	not valid	valid	1
	Criterion validity	not tested	not valid	valid	-
Reliability	Internal consistency	not tested	not consistent	consistent	-
	Reproducibility	not tested	not reproducible	reproducible	-
	Responsiveness	not tested	not responsive	responsive	-
				Subtotal	1

Clinical utility ●●●● (4/4)

	0 points	1 point	2 points	points
Patient friendliness	limited	moderate	strong	2
Clinician friendliness	limited	moderate	strong	2
			Subtotal	4

Total (out of 10) ●●●●●○○○○○ **5**

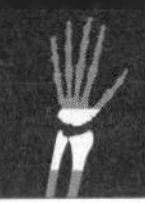

9. Gartland and Werley scoring system (modified by Sarmiento) (1951)

Source: Gartland JJ Jr., Werley CW (1951) Evaluation of healed Colles' fractures.
J Bone Joint Surg Am; 33-A:895–907.

Content

Type Clinician based outcome
Scale 4 subscales (6 items):

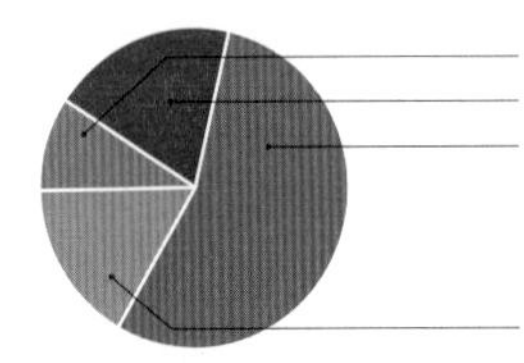

Residual deformity (3 points)
Subjective evaluation (6 points)
Objective evaluation
- Loss of range of motion (15 points)
- Pain (1 point)
- Loss of grip strength (1 point)

Complications (5 points)

Interpretation

Excellent: 0–2 points
Good: 3–8 points
Fair: 9–20 points
Poor: > 20 points

Validation

Outcomes validated against

- Functional index

Patient population tested in	Validity	Reliability	Responsiveness
Patients with fractures of the distal radius (60 years; 20% male)	+	not tested	not tested

Validation study:

Porter ML, Stockley I (1951) Functional index: a numerical expression of post-traumatic wrist function. Injury; 16:188–192.

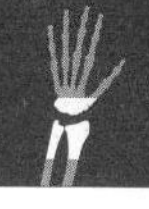

Methodological evaluation ●○○○○○ (1/6)

		no score	0 points	1 point	points
Validity	Content validity	not tested	not valid	valid	-
	Construct validity	not tested	not valid	valid	1
	Criterion validity	not tested	not valid	valid	-
Reliability	Internal consistency	not tested	not consistent	consistent	-
	Reproducibility	not tested	not reproducible	reproducible	-
	Responsiveness	not tested	not responsive	responsive	-
				Subtotal	1

Clinical utility ●●●○ (3/4)

	0 points	1 point	2 points	points
Patient friendliness	limited	moderate	strong	2
Clinician friendliness	limited	moderate	strong	1
			Subtotal	3

Total (out of 10) ●●●●○○○○○○ **4**

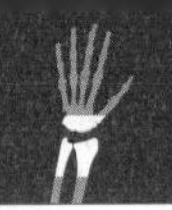

10. Green and O'Brien (1978)

Source: Green DP, O'Brien ET (1978) Open reduction of carpal dislocations: indications and operative techniques.
J Hand Surg [Am], 3:250–265.
Source modified Green and O'Brien: Cooney WP, Bussey R, Dobyns JH, Linscheid RL (1987) Difficult wrist fractures. Perilunate fracture-dislocations of the wrist.
Clin Orthop; (214):136–147.

Content

Type Clinician based outcome
Scale 5 subscales (5 items):

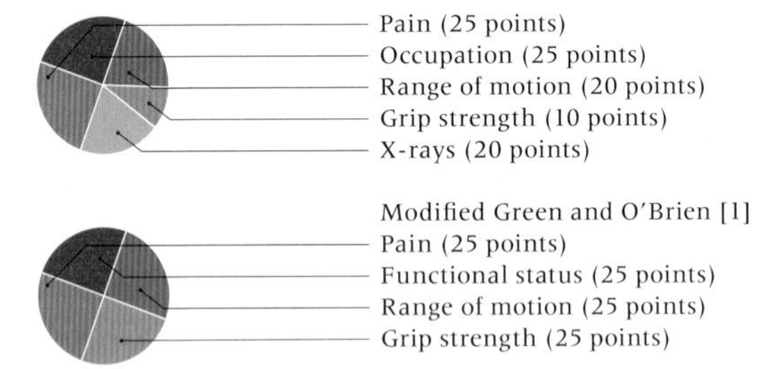

Interpretation

Minimum score: 0 points
Maximum score: 100 points

The higher the score, the higher the function.

Validation

No validation studies were identified.

Patient population tested in	Validity	Reliability	Responsiveness
Not applicable			

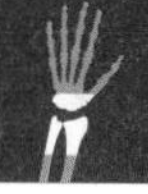

Methodological evaluation

○○○○○○ (0/6)

		no score	0 points	1 point	points
Validity	Content validity	not tested	not valid	valid	-
	Construct validity	not tested	not valid	valid	-
	Criterion validity	not tested	not valid	valid	-
Reliability	Internal consistency	not tested	not consistent	consistent	-
	Reproducibility	not tested	not reproducible	reproducible	-
	Responsiveness	not tested	not responsive	responsive	-
				Subtotal	-

Clinical utility

●●●○ (3/4)

	0 points	1 point	2 points	points
Patient friendliness	limited	moderate	strong	2
Clinician friendliness	limited	moderate	strong	1
			Subtotal	3

Total (out of 10) 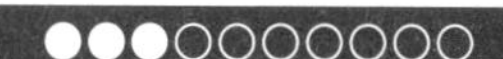 **3**

11. Hand functional index (1988)

Source: Kalla AA, Kotze TJ, Meyers OL, Parkyn ND (1988) Clinical assessment of disease activity in rheumatoid arthritis: evaluation of a functional test.
Ann Rheum Dis; 47:773–779.

Content

Type Clinician based outcome
Scale 3 subscales (9 items):

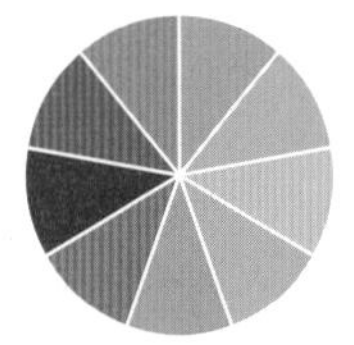

9 tasks measuring functional range of motion for each wrist/hand.
Tasks are not equally weighted and range between 2 to 3 possible points.

Interpretation

Each hand/wrist scored separately.

Minimum score: 0 points
Maximum score: 21 points

The higher the score, the lower the function.

Validation

Outcomes validated against

- Keitel function test

Patient population tested in	Validity	Reliability	Responsiveness
Patients with rheumatoid arthritis (38 years; 29% male)	+	not tested	not tested

Validation study:

Kalla AA, Kotze TJ, Meyers OL, Parkyn ND (1988) Clinical assessment of disease activity in rheumatoid arthritis: evaluation of a functional test. Ann Rheum Dis; 47:773–779.

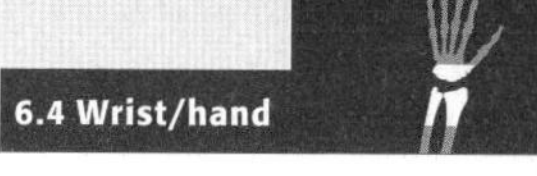

Methodological evaluation

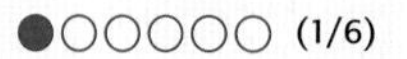 (1/6)

		no score	0 points	1 point	points
Validity	Content validity	not tested	not valid	valid	-
	Construct validity	not tested	not valid	valid	1
	Criterion validity	not tested	not valid	valid	-
Reliability	Internal consistency	not tested	not consistent	consistent	-
	Reproducibility	not tested	not reproducible	reproducible	-
	Responsiveness	not tested	not responsive	responsive	-
				Subtotal	**1**

Clinical utility

●●○○ (2/4)

	0 points	1 point	2 points	points
Patient friendliness	limited	moderate	strong	2
Clinician friendliness	limited	moderate	strong	0
			Subtotal	**2**

Total (out of 10) 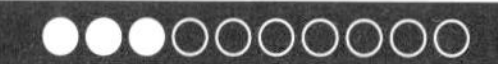 **3**

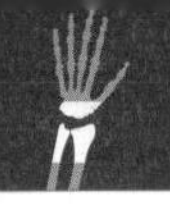

12. Hospital for Special Surgery wrist scoring system (HSS) (1990)

Source: Figgie MP, Ranawat CS, Inglis AE, Sobel M, Figgie HE 3rd (1990) Trispherical total wrist arthroplasty in rheumatoid arthritis. J Hand Surg [Am]; 15:217–223.

Content

Type Clinician based outcome
Scale 3 subscales (4 items):

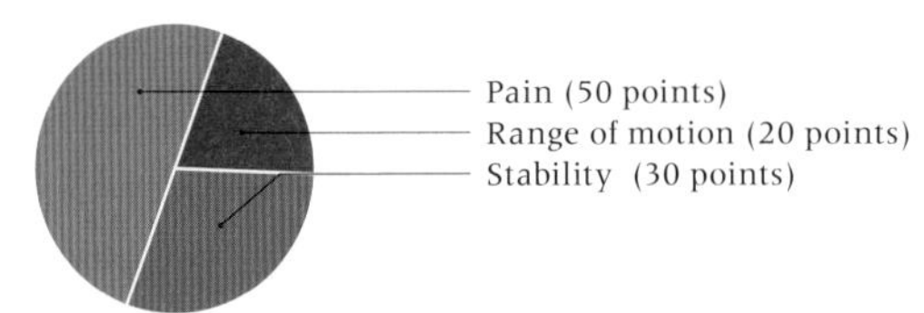

Interpretation

Excellent: 90–100 points
Good: 80–89 points
Fair: 70–79 points
Failure: < 60 points

Validation

No validation studies were identified.

Patient population tested in	Validity	Reliability	Responsiveness
Not applicable			

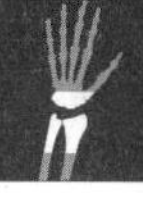

Methodological evaluation

○○○○○○ (0/6)

		no score	0 points	1 point	points
Validity	Content validity	not tested	not valid	valid	-
	Construct validity	not tested	not valid	valid	-
	Criterion validity	not tested	not valid	valid	-
Reliability	Internal consistency	not tested	not consistent	consistent	-
	Reproducibility	not tested	not reproducible	reproducible	-
	Responsiveness	not tested	not responsive	responsive	-
				Subtotal	-

Clinical utility

●●●● (4/4)

	0 points	1 point	2 points	points
Patient friendliness	limited	moderate	strong	2
Clinician friendliness	limited	moderate	strong	2
			Subtotal	4

Total (out of 10)

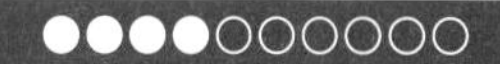

4

13. Kapandji index (1987)

Source: Kapandji A (1987) [Proposal for a clinical score for flexion-extension of the long fingers].
Ann Chir Main; 6:288–294.

Content

Type Clinician based outcome
Scale 3 subscales (3 items):

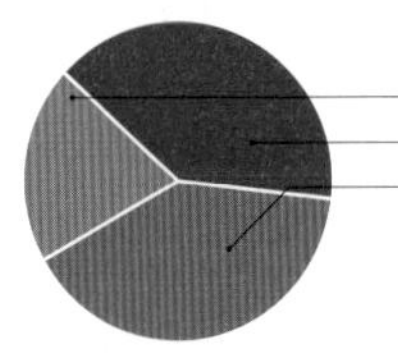

Opposition of the thumb (10 points)
Flexion of each long finger (20 points)
Finger extension (20 points)

Interpretation

Minimum score: 0 points
Maximum score: 50 points
The higher the score, the higher the function.

Validation

Outcomes validated against [1]

- Hand function index
- Finger mobility
- Grip and pinch strength
- Cochin scale
- VAS for pain
- Larsen radiological grading

Patient population tested in	Validity	Reliability	Responsiveness
Patients with rheumatoid arthritis of the hand scheduled for surgery (57 years; 14% male) [1]	not tested	+	not tested
Patients with rheumatoid arthritis of the hand scheduled for surgery (54 years; 16% male) [1]	+	not tested	-
Patients with rheumatoid arthritis of the hand scheduled for surgery (54 years; 16% male) [2]	not tested	not tested	-

Validation studies:

[1] Lefevre-Colau MM, Poiraudeau S, Oberlin C, et al (2003) Reliability, validity, and responsiveness of the modified Kapandji index for assessment of functional mobility of the rheumatoid hand. Arch Phys Med Rehabil; 84:1032–1038.

[2] Lefevre-Colau MM, Poiraudeau S, Fermanian J, et al (2001) Responsiveness of the Cochin rheumatoid hand disability scale after surgery. Rheumatology (Oxford); 84:843–850.

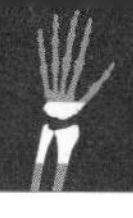

Methodological evaluation

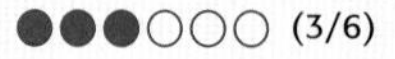 (3/6)

		no score	0 points	1 point	points
Validity	Content validity	not tested	not valid	valid	1
	Construct validity	not tested	not valid	valid	1
	Criterion validity	not tested	not valid	valid	-
Reliability	Internal consistency	not tested	not consistent	consistent	-
	Reproducibility	not tested	not reproducible	reproducible	1
	Responsiveness	not tested	not responsive	responsive	0
				Subtotal	**3**

Clinical utility

●●●● (4/4)

	0 points	1 point	2 points	points
Patient friendliness	limited	moderate	strong	2
Clinician friendliness	limited	moderate	strong	2
			Subtotal	**4**

Total (out of 10)  **7**

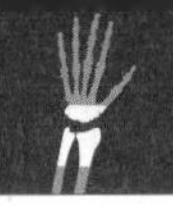

14. Lamberta and Clayton wrist score (1980)

Source: Lamberta FJ, Ferlic DC, Clayton ML (1980) Volz total wrist arthroplasty in rheumatoid arthritis: a preliminary report. J Hand Surg [Am]; 5:245–252.

Content

Type Clinician based outcome
Scale 5 subscales (5 items)

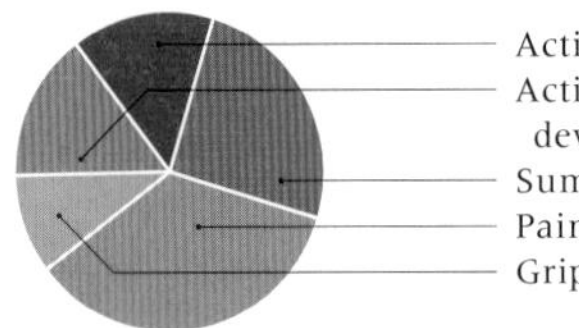

Interpretation

Minimum score: 0 points
Maximum score: 100 points

The higher the score, the higher the function.

Validation

No validation studies were identified.

Patient population tested in	Validity	Reliability	Responsiveness
Not applicable			

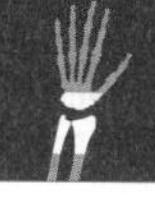

Methodological evaluation

○○○○○○ (0/6)

		no score	0 points	1 point	points
Validity	Content validity	not tested	not valid	valid	-
	Construct validity	not tested	not valid	valid	-
	Criterion validity	not tested	not valid	valid	-
Reliability	Internal consistency	not tested	not consistent	consistent	-
	Reproducibility	not tested	not reproducible	reproducible	-
	Responsiveness	not tested	not responsive	responsive	-
				Subtotal	0

Clinical utility

●●●○ (3/4)

	0 points	1 point	2 points	points
Patient friendliness	limited	moderate	strong	2
Clinician friendliness	limited	moderate	strong	1
			Subtotal	3

Total (out of 10) 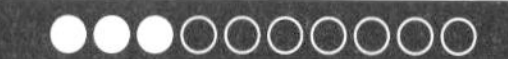 **3**

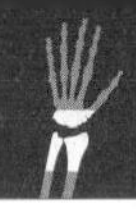

15. MacBain hand function test (1970)

Source: MacBain KP (1970) Assessment of function in the rheumatoid hand.
Can J Occup Ther; 37:95–103.

Content

Type Clinician based outcome
Scale 3 subscales (7 items):

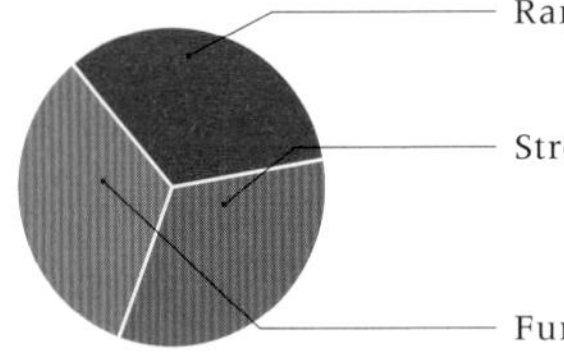

Range of motion
- Fingers to palm
- Opposition

Strength
- Power grip
- Pinch
- Finger hook strength

Functional tasks
- Applied strength (play dough, pour cup, kettle)
- Precision (buttons, pin, lacing, door, coins)

Interpretation

Each task is scored and given one of the following grades based on normative values established from a control group:

- Normal
- Good
- Fair
- Poor

Validation

No validation studies were identified.

Patient population tested in	Validity	Reliability	Responsiveness
Not applicable			

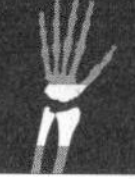

Methodological evaluation

○○○○○○ (0/6)

		no score	0 points	1 point	points
Validity	Content validity	not tested	not valid	valid	-
	Construct validity	not tested	not valid	valid	-
	Criterion validity	not tested	not valid	valid	-
Reliability	Internal consistency	not tested	not consistent	consistent	-
	Reproducibility	not tested	not reproducible	reproducible	-
	Responsiveness	not tested	not responsive	responsive	-
				Subtotal	-

Clinical utility

●●●● (4/4)

	0 points	1 point	2 points	points
Patient friendliness	limited	moderate	strong	2
Clinician friendliness	limited	moderate	strong	2
			Subtotal	4

Total (out of 10) 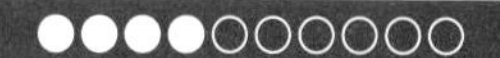 **4**

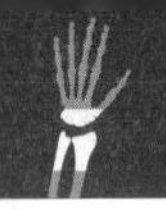

16. Michigan Hand outcomes Questionnaire (MHQ) (1998)

Source: Chung KC, Pillsbury MS, Walters MR, Hayward RA (1998) Reliability and validity testing of the Michigan Hand Outcomes Questionnaire.
J Hand Surg [Am]; 23:575–587.

Content

Type Patient reported outcome
Scale 6 subscales (65 items):

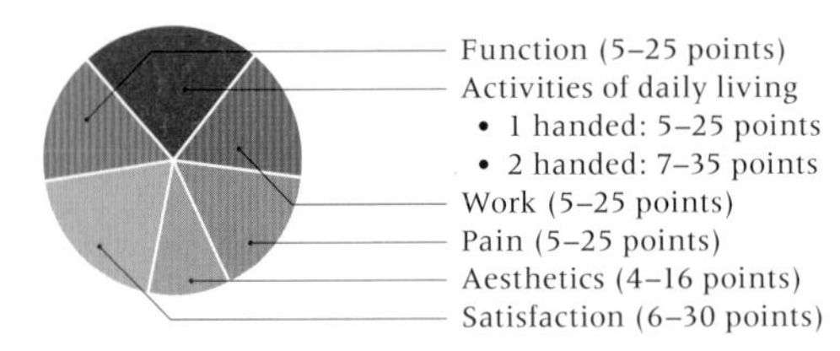

Interpretation

Each subscale scored separately and normalized to 100.
Average score of the six subscales = total MHQ score.

Validation

Outcomes validated against [1]

- SF-12

Patient population tested in	Validity	Reliability	Responsiveness
Patients with hand disorders (45 years; 53% male) [1]	+	+	not tested
Patients with chronic hand disorders (48 years; 57% male) [2]	not tested	not tested	+

Validation studies:

[1] Chung KC, Pillsbury MS, Walters MR, et al (1998) Reliability and validity testing of the Michigan Hand Outcomes Questionnaire. J Hand Surg [Am]; 23:575–587.
[2] Chung KC, Hamill JB, Walters MR, et al (1999) The Michigan Hand Outcomes Questionnaire (MHQ): assessment of responsiveness to clinical change. Ann Plast Surg; 42:619–622.

Methodological evaluation

●●●●●○ (5/6)

		no score	0 points	1 point	points
Validity	Content validity	not tested	not valid	valid	1
	Construct validity	not tested	not valid	valid	1
	Criterion validity	not tested	not valid	valid	-
Reliability	Internal consistency	not tested	not consistent	consistent	1
	Reproducibility	not tested	not reproducible	reproducible	1
	Responsiveness	not tested	not responsive	responsive	1
				Subtotal	**5**

Clinical utility

●●○○ (2/4)

	0 points	1 point	2 points	points
Patient friendliness	limited	moderate	strong	2
Clinician friendliness	limited	moderate	strong	0
			Subtotal	**2**

Total (out of 10) ●●●●●●●○○○ **7**

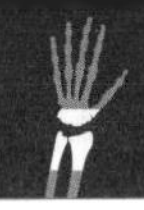

17. New York Orthopedic Hospital wrist rating system (1993)

Source: Kaempffe FA, Wheeler DR, Peimer CA, Hvisdak KS, Ceravolo J, Senall J (1993) Severe fractures of the distal radius: effect of amount and duration of external fixator distraction on outcome. J Hand Surg [Am]; 18:33–41.

Content

Type Clinician based outcome
Scale 5 subscales:

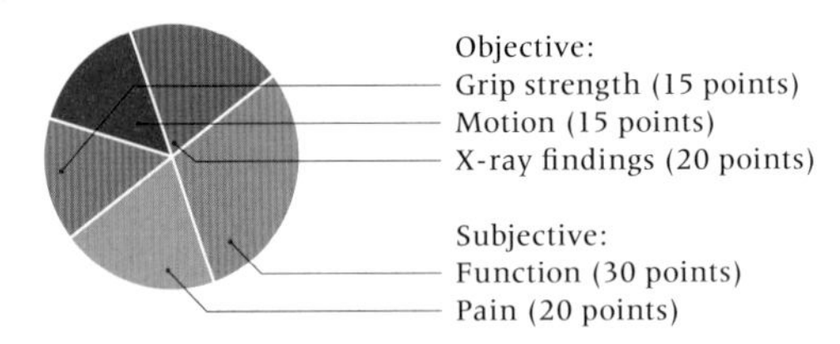

Interpretation

Excellent: 90–100 points
Good: 70–89 points
Fair: 55–69 points
Poor: < 55 points

Validation

No validation studies were identified.

Patient population tested in	Validity	Reliability	Responsiveness
Not applicable			

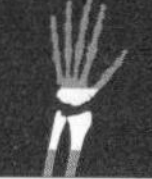

Methodological evaluation

○○○○○○ (0/6)

		no score	0 points	1 point	points
Validity	Content validity	not tested	not valid	valid	-
	Construct validity	not tested	not valid	valid	-
	Criterion validity	not tested	not valid	valid	-
Reliability	Internal consistency	not tested	not consistent	consistent	-
	Reproducibility	not tested	not reproducible	reproducible	-
	Responsiveness	not tested	not responsive	responsive	-
				Subtotal	-

Clinical utility

●●●● (4/4)

	0 points	1 point	2 points	points
Patient friendliness	limited	moderate	strong	2
Clinician friendliness	limited	moderate	strong	2
			Subtotal	4

Total (out of 10) 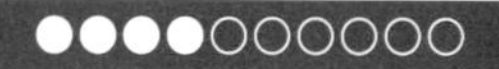 **4**

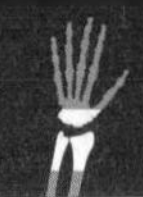

18. Patient focused wrist outcome (2003)

Source: Bialocerkowski AE, Grimmer KA, Bain GI (2003)
Development of a patient-focused wrist outcome instrument.
Hand Clin; 19:437–448.

Content

Type Patient reported outcome
Scale 2 subscales (30 items):

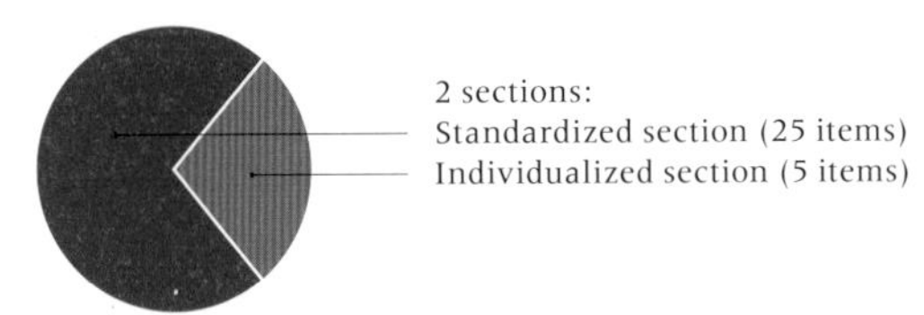

Standardized section:
25 items pertaining to performing activities of daily living.

Four possible responses to each question:
- Yes, I have difficulty with this activity.
- No, I don't have difficulty with this activity.
- I haven't tried to perform this activity, but I would normally perform it.
- I won't normally perform this activity.

Individualized section:
Patient is able to nominate up to 5 additional activities not in the standardized section that are important yet difficult to perform.

Individuals rate the level of difficulty on a 5-point Likert scale. (1 = no difficulty; 5 = cannot do it at all) and the importance of each activity on a 5-point Likert scale (1 = no importance at all; 5 = essential).

Interpretation

The two sections are scored separately.

Standardized section:
Sum of the number of "yes" responses.
Minimum score: 0 points
Maximum score: 25 points

Individualized section:
Sum of difficulty and importance scores
Minimum: 10 points
Maximum: 50 points

The higher the score, the lower the function

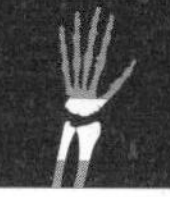

Validation

Outcomes validated against [1]
- Glasgow pain questionnaire

Patient population tested in	Validity	Reliability	Responsiveness
Patients who had sustained a distal radius fracture (61.8 years; 15% male) [1]	+	not tested	+
Patients with unilateral, non-systemic, musculoskeletal wrist disorders (age and sex NR) [2]	+	+	not tested

Validation studies:

[1] Bialocerkowski AE, Grimmer KA, Bain GI (2003) Validity of the patient-focused wrist outcome instrument: do impairments represent functional ability? Hand Clin; 19:449–455.
[2] Bialocerkowski AE, Grimmer KA, Bain GI: Development of a patient-focused wrist outcome instrument. Hand Clin; 19:437–448.

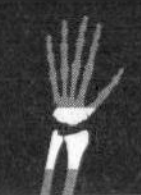

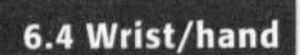

18. Patient focused wrist outcome (2003)

Details see previous pages.

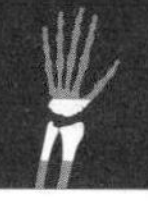

Methodological evaluation

●●●●○○ (4/6)

		no score	0 points	1 point	points
Validity	Content validity	not tested	not valid	**valid**	1
	Construct validity	not tested	not valid	**valid**	1
	Criterion validity	**not tested**	not valid	valid	-
Reliability	Internal consistency	**not tested**	not consistent	consistent	-
	Reproducibility	not tested	not reproducible	**reproducible**	1
	Responsiveness	not tested	not responsive	**responsive**	1
				Subtotal	**4**

Clinical utility

●●○○ (2/4)

	0 points	1 point	2 points	points
Patient friendliness	**limited**	moderate	strong	0
Clinician friendliness	limited	moderate	**strong**	2
			Subtotal	**2**

Total (out of 10) ●●●●●●○○○○ **6**

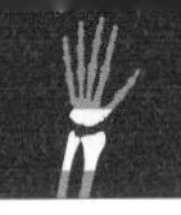

19. Patient Outcomes of Surgery-Hand/Arm (POS-Hand/Arm) (2004)

Source: Cano SJ, Browne JP, Lamping DL, Roberts AH, McGrouther DA, Black NA (2004) The Patient Outcomes of Surgery-Hand/Arm (POS-Hand/Arm): a new patient-based outcome measure. J Hand Surg [Br]; 29:477–485.

Content

Type Patient reported outcome
Scales 33 items:

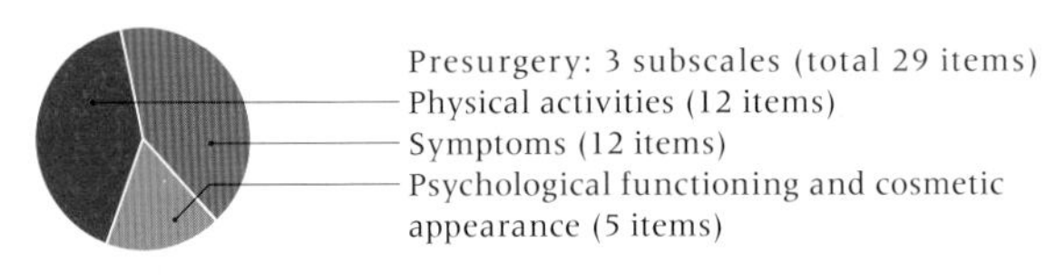

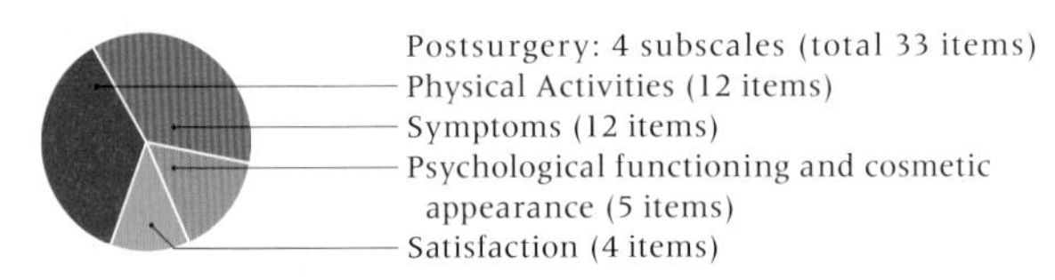

Interpretation

Each scale normalized to 100 and scored separately.

The higher the score, the higher the function.

Validation

Outcomes validated against

- SF-36
- DASH
- MHQ

Patient population tested in	Validity	Reliability	Responsiveness
Patients with hand/arm conditions (57 years; 47% male)	+	+	+

Validation study:

Cano SJ, Browne JP, Lamping DL, et al (2004) The Patient Outcomes of Surgery-Hand/Arm (POS-Hand/Arm): a new patient-based outcome measure. J Hand Surg [Br]; 29:477–485.

19. Patient Outcomes of Surgery-Hand/Arm (POS-Hand/Arm) (2004)

Methodological evaluation

(5/6)

		no score	0 points	1 point	points
Validity	Content validity	not tested	not valid	**valid**	1
Validity	Construct validity	not tested	not valid	**valid**	1
Validity	Criterion validity	**not tested**	not valid	valid	-
Reliability	Internal consistency	not tested	not consistent	**consistent**	1
Reliability	Reproducibility	not tested	not reproducible	**reproducible**	1
	Responsiveness	not tested	not responsive	**responsive**	1
				Subtotal	**5**

Clinical utility

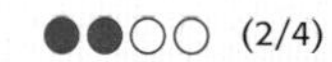
(2/4)

	0 points	1 point	2 points	points
Patient friendliness	**limited**	moderate	strong	0
Clinician friendliness	limited	moderate	**strong**	2
			Subtotal	**2**

Total (out of 10)

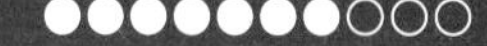

7

20. Patient Rated Wrist Evaluation (PRWE) (1998)

Source: MacDermid JC, Turgeon T, Richards RS, Beadle M, Roth JH (1998) Patient rating of wrist pain and disability: a reliable and valid measurement tool.
J Orthop Trauma; 12:577–586.

Content

Type Patient reported outcome
Scale 2 subscales (15 items):

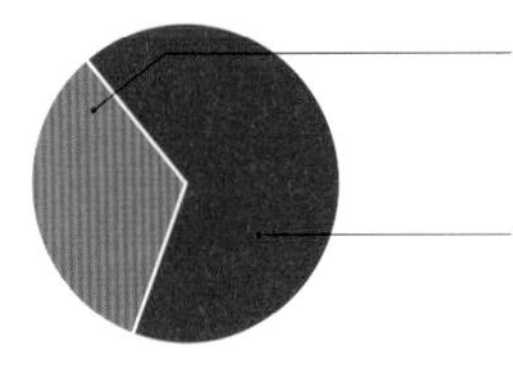

Pain (5 items):
- When at rest
- When moving wrist or lifting
- When at worst

Function (10 items):
- When performing various specific activities of daily living
- When doing work (job and home), recreation, and personal care

Interpretation

Minimum score: 0 points
Maximum score: 100 points

The higher the score, the lower the function.

Validation

Outcomes validated against [1]

- Range of motion, grip strength, dexterity testing
- SF-36
- Expected changes in pain and disability

Patient population tested in	Validity	Reliability	Responsiveness
Patients with Colles fractures (50 years; 31% male) or scaphoid nonunion (34 years; 97% male) [1]	+	not tested	not tested
Patient with acute and treated Colles fractures (60 years; 36% male and 45 years; 33% male, respectively) and scaphoid nonunion (34 years; 97% male) [1]	not tested	+	not tested
Patients with wrist fractures or carpal instabilities (age range, 21–75 years; 43% male) [2]	not tested	not tested	+
Patients with distal radius fractures (53 years; 37% male) [3]	not tested	not tested	+
Chinese (n=21) or English (n=30) speaking patients with distal radius fracture (age NR; 73% male) [4]	not tested	+	not tested

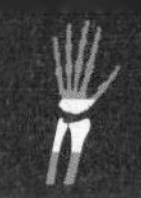

Validation (cont)

Validation studies:

[1] MacDermid JC, Turgeon T, Richards RS, et al (1998) Patient rating of wrist pain and disability: a reliable and valid measurement tool. J Orthop Trauma; 12:577–586.

[2] MacDermid JC, Tottenham V (2004) Responsiveness of the disability of the arm, shoulder, and hand (DASH) and patient-rated wrist/hand evaluation (PRWHE) in evaluating change after hand therapy. J Hand Ther; 17:18–23.

[3] MacDermid JC, Richards RS, Donner A, et al (2000) Responsiveness of the short form-36, disability of the arm, shoulder, and hand questionnaire, patient-rated wrist evaluation, and physical impairment measurements in evaluating recovery after a distal radius fracture. J Hand Surg [Am]; 25:330–340.

[4] Xu W, Seow C (2003) Chinese version of patient rated wrist evaluation (PRWE): cross cultural adaptation and reliability evaluation. Ann Acad Med Singapore; 32(5Suppl):48–49.

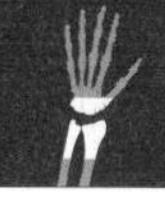

Methodological evaluation

●●●●●● (6/6)

		no score	0 points	1 point	points
Validity	Content validity	not tested	not valid	valid	1
	Construct validity	not tested	not valid	valid	1
	Criterion validity	not tested	not valid	valid	1
Reliability	Internal consistency	not tested	not consistent	consistent	1
	Reproducibility	not tested	not reproducible	reproducible	1
	Responsiveness	not tested	not responsive	responsive*	1
				Subtotal	6

* Chinese version only.

Clinical utility

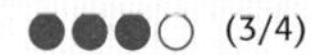

(3/4)

	0 points	1 point	2 points	points
Patient friendliness	limited	moderate	strong	1
Clinician friendliness	limited	moderate	strong	2
			Subtotal	3

Total (out of 10)

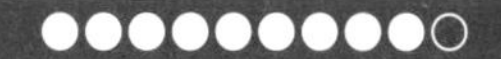

9

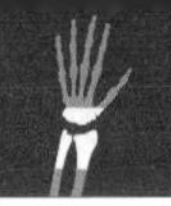

21. Quick DASH (1996)

Source: King GJ, Richards RR, Zuckerman JD, Blasier R, Dillman C, Friedman RJ, Gartsman GM, Iannotti JP, Murnahan JP, Mow VC, Woo SL (1999) A standardized method for assessment of elbow function. Research Committee, American Shoulder and Elbow Surgeons. J Shoulder Elbow Surg, 8:351–354.

Content

3 modules
Module 1: ability to perform (required)
Scale 5 subscales (11 items):

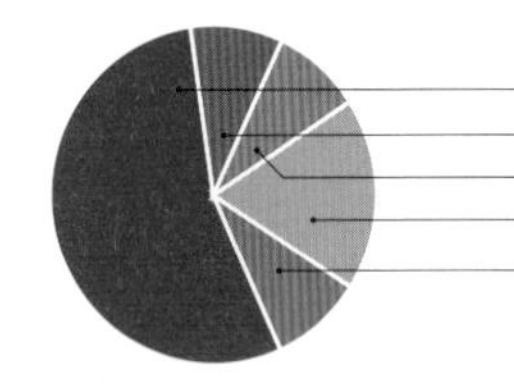

Activities of daily living (30 points)
Social activities (5 points)
Work activities (5 points)
Symptoms (10 points)
Sleeping (5 points)

Module 2: ability to perform sports/performing arts (optional)
Scale
Sports/performing arts (20 points)

Module 3: ability to perform work (optional)
Scale
Work (20 points)

Interpretation
Each module is scored separately.

Normalized to 100:
[(Sum of responses / number of completed responses) – 1] × 25 = Quick DASH score

Minimum score: 0 points
Maximum score: 100 points

The higher the score, the lower the function.

Validation

No validation studies were identified.

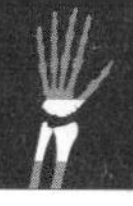

Methodological evaluation

○○○○○○ (0/6)

		no score	0 points	1 point	points
Validity	Content validity	not tested	not valid	valid	-
	Construct validity	not tested	not valid	valid	-
	Criterion validity	not tested	not valid	valid	-
Reliability	Internal consistency	not tested	not consistent	consistent	-
	Reproducibility	not tested	not reproducible	reproducible	-
	Responsiveness	not tested	not responsive	responsive	-
				Subtotal	-

Clinical utility

●●●○ (3/4)

	0 points	1 point	2 points	points
Patient friendliness	limited	moderate	strong	1
Clinician friendliness	limited	moderate	strong	2
			Subtotal	3

Total (out of 10) ●●●○○○○○○○ **3**

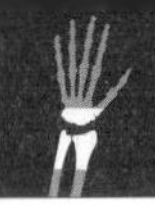

22. Sequential Occupational Dexterity Assessment (SODA) (1996)

Source: van Lankveld W, van't Pad Bosch P, Bakker J, Terwindt S, Franssen M, van Riel P (1996) Sequential occupational dexterity assessment (SODA): a new test to measure hand disability. J Hand Ther; 9:27–32.

Content

Type Clinician based outcome
Scale 1 subscale (12 items):

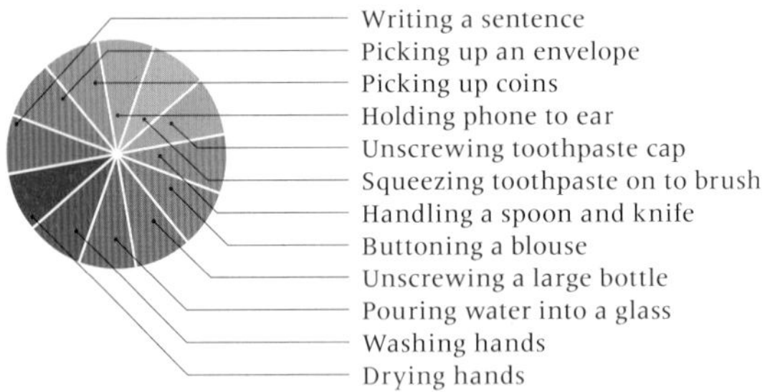

Interpretation

Minimum score: 0 points; maximum score: 108 points
The higher the score, the higher the function.

Validation

Outcomes validated against

- Range of motion of wrist
- Mobility of fingers
- Grip strength
- Self-reported dexterity
- Pain

Patient population tested in	Validity	Reliability	Responsiveness
Patients with classic or definite Rheumatoid arthritis (60.3 years; 64% male)	not tested	+	not tested
Patients who had undergone hand surgery for a variety of problems (54.6 years; 71% male)	not tested	not tested	+
Patients with classic or definite Rheumatoid arthritis (54.5 years; 34% male)	+	+	not tested

Validation study:

van Lankveld W, van't Pad Bosch P, Bakker J, et al (1996) Sequential occupational dexterity assessment (SODA). J Hand Ther; 9:27–32.

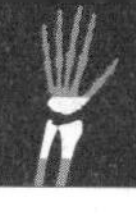

Methodological evaluation

●●●●●○ (5/6)

		no score	0 points	1 point	points
Validity	Content validity	not tested	not valid	valid	1
	Construct validity	not tested	not valid	valid	1
	Criterion validity	not tested	not valid	valid	-
Reliability	Internal consistency	not tested	not consistent	consistent	1
	Reproducibility	not tested	not reproducible	reproducible	1
	Responsiveness	not tested	not responsive	responsive	1
				Subtotal	**5**

Clinical utility

●●●● (4/4)

	0 points	1 point	2 points	points
Patient friendliness	limited	moderate	strong	2
Clinician friendliness	limited	moderate	strong	2
			Subtotal	**4**

Total (out of 10) 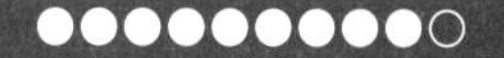 **9**

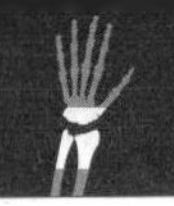

23. Upper extremity function scale (1997)

Source: Pransky G, Feuerstein M, Himmelstein J, Katz JN, Vickers-Lahti M (1997) Measuring functional outcomes in work-related upper extremity disorders. Development and validation of the Upper Extremity Function Scale.
J Occup Environ Med; 39:1195–1202.

Content

Type Patient reported outcome
Scale 8 items:

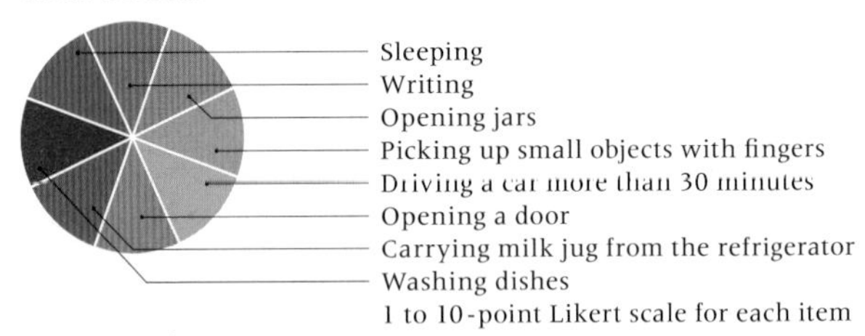

1 to 10-point Likert scale for each item

Interpretation

Minimum score: 8 points
Maximum score: 80 points
The higher the score, the lower the function.

Validation

Outcomes validated against

- Physical findings (grip, pinch, and Phalen's test)
- Duration of symptoms
- Working status
- Arthritis Impact Measurement Scale

Patient population tested in	Validity	Reliability	Responsiveness
Patients with work related upper extremity disorders (38 years; 34% male)	+	+	+
Patients with carpal tunnel syndrome (46 years; 33% male)			

Validation study:

Pransky G, Feuerstein M, Himmelstein J, et al (1997) Measuring functional outcomes in work-related upper extremity disorders. Development and validation of the Upper Extremity Function Scale. J Occup Environ Med; 39:1195–1202.

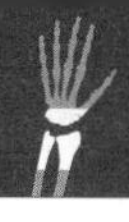

Methodological evaluation

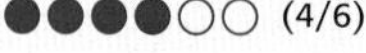 (4/6)

		no score	0 points	1 point	points
Validity	Content validity	not tested	not valid	valid	1
	Construct validity	not tested	not valid	valid	1
	Criterion validity	not tested	not valid	valid	-
Reliability	Internal consistency	not tested	not consistent	consistent	1
	Reproducibility	not tested	not reproducible	reproducible	-
	Responsiveness	not tested	not responsive	responsive	1
				Subtotal	**4**

Clinical utility

●●●● (4/4)

	0 points	1 point	2 points	points
Patient friendliness	limited	moderate	strong	2
Clinician friendliness	limited	moderate	strong	2
			Subtotal	**4**

Total (out of 10) 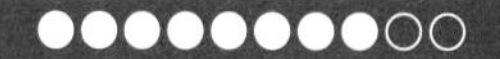 **8**

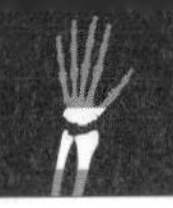

24. Wrightington wrist function score (1998)

Source: Van Den Abbeele KL, Loh YC, Stanley JK, Trail IA (1998) Early results of a modified Brunelli procedure for scapholunate instability. J Hand Surg [Br]; 23:258–261.

Content

Type Clinician based outcome
Scale 8 items:

8 tasks graded from 1 (normal) to 4 (unable to perform):

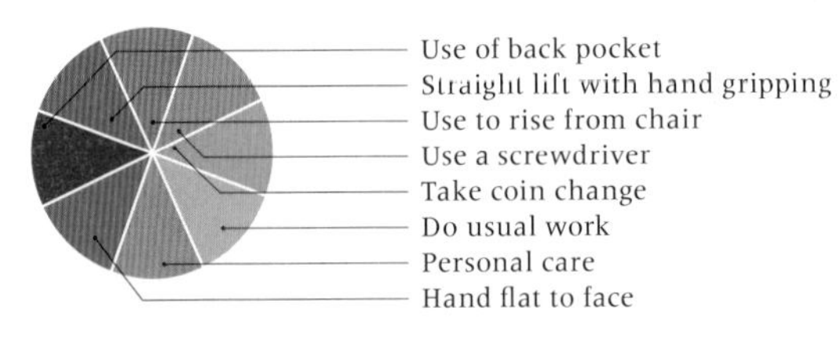

Interpretation

Minimum score: 8 points
Maximum score: 32 points

The higher the score the, the lower the function.

Validation

No validation studies were identified.

Patient population tested in	Validity	Reliability	Responsiveness
Not applicable			

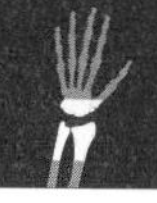

Methodological evaluation

○○○○○○ (0/6)

		no score	0 points	1 point	points
Validity	Content validity	not tested	not valid	valid	-
	Construct validity	not tested	not valid	valid	-
	Criterion validity	not tested	not valid	valid	-
Reliability	Internal consistency	not tested	not consistent	consistent	-
	Reproducibility	not tested	not reproducible	reproducible	-
	Responsiveness	not tested	not responsive	responsive	-
				Subtotal	-

Clinical utility

●●●● (4/4)

	0 points	1 point	2 points	points
Patient friendliness	limited	moderate	strong	2
Clinician friendliness	limited	moderate	strong	2
			Subtotal	4

Total (out of 10) 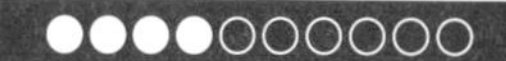 **4**

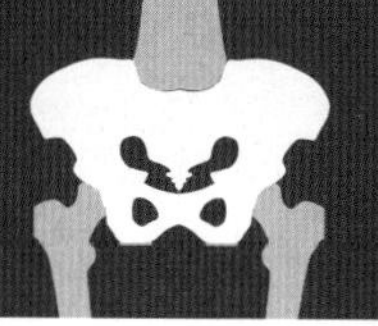

6.5 Pelvis

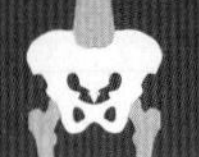

1. Iowa pelvic score (1996)

Source: Templeman D, Goulet J, Duwelius PJ, Olson S, Davidson M (1996) Internal fixation of displaced fractures of the sacrum. Clin Orthop; (329):180–185.

Content

Type Patient reported outcome
Scale 6 subscales (25 items):

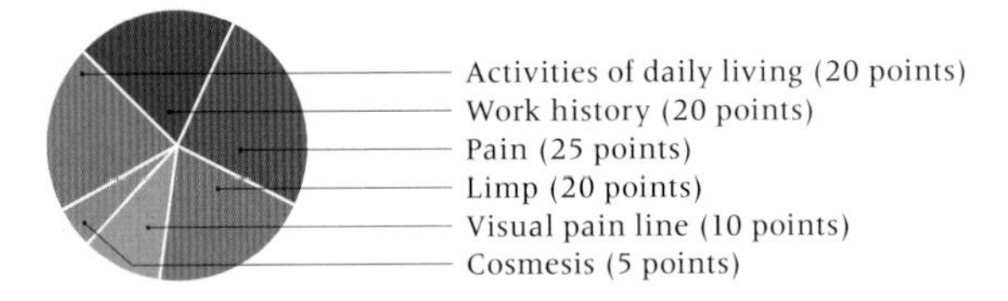

Interpretation

Original not designed with qualitative grades:
Excellent: 85–100 points
Good: 70–84 points
Fair: 55–69 points
Poor: < 55 points

Validation

Outcomes validated against

- SF-36

Patient population tested in	Validity	Reliability	Responsiveness
Pelvic ring injury (37 years; 61% male)	+	not tested	not tested

Validation study:

Nepola JV, Trenhaile SW, Miranda MA, et al (1999) Vertical shear injuries: is there a relationship between residual displacement and functional outcome? J Trauma; 46:1024–1029.

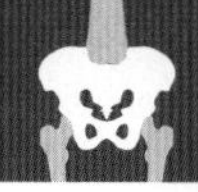

Methodological evaluation

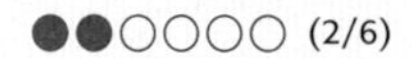 (2/6)

		no score	0 points	1 point	points
Validity	Content validity	not tested	not valid	valid	1
	Construct validity	not tested	not valid	valid	-
	Criterion validity	not tested	not valid	valid	1
Reliability	Internal consistency	not tested	not consistent	consistent	-
	Reproducibility	not tested	not reproducible	reproducible	-
	Responsiveness	not tested	not responsive	responsive	-
				Subtotal	**2**

Clinical utility

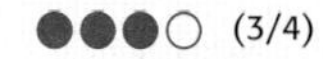 (3/4)

	0 points	1 point	2 points	points
Patient friendliness	limited	moderate	strong	2
Clinician friendliness	limited	moderate	strong	1
			Subtotal	**3**

Total (out of 10) 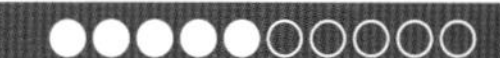 **5**

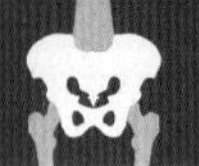

2. Majeed pelvic score (1989)

Source: Majeed SA (1989) Grading the outcome of pelvic fractures. J Bone Joint Surg Br; 71:304–306.

Other versions available: Dutch.

Content

Type Patient reported outcome
Scale 5 subscales (7 items):

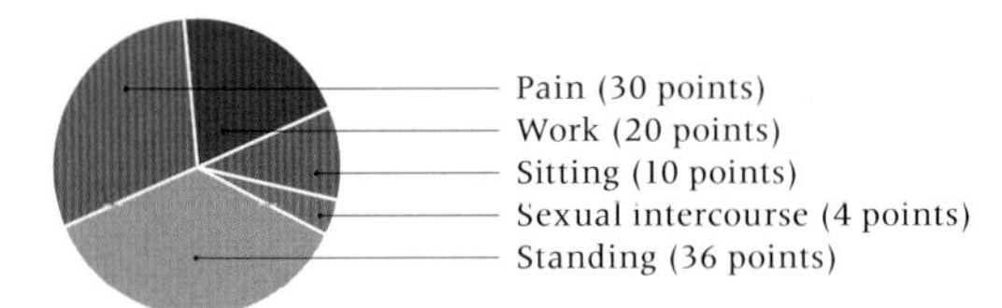

Interpretation

Working
Excellent: > 85 points
Good: 70–84 points
Fair: 55–69 points
Poor: < 55 points

Not working
Excellent: > 70 points
Good: 55–69 points
Fair: 45–54 points
Poor: < 45 points

Validation

Outcomes validated against

- SF-36

Patient population tested in	Validity	Reliability	Responsiveness
Pelvic ring injury (35 years; 70% male)	+	not tested	not tested

Validation study:
Van den Bosch EW, Van der Kleyn R, Hogervorst M, et al (1999) Functional outcome of internal fixation for pelvic ring fractures. J Trauma; 47:365–371.

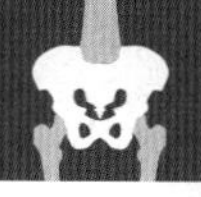

Methodological evaluation

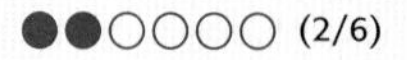
(2/6)

		no score	0 points	1 point	points
Validity	Content validity	not tested	not valid	**valid**	1
	Construct validity	**not tested**	not valid	valid	-
	Criterion validity	not tested	not valid	**valid**	1
Reliability	Internal consistency	**not tested**	not consistent	consistent	-
	Reproducibility	**not tested**	not reproducible	reproducible	-
	Responsiveness	**not tested**	not responsive	responsive	-
				Subtotal	**2**

Clinical utility

●●●○ (3/4)

	0 points	1 point	2 points	points
Patient friendliness	limited	moderate	**strong**	2
Clinician friendliness	limited	**moderate**	strong	1
			Subtotal	**3**

Total (out of 10)

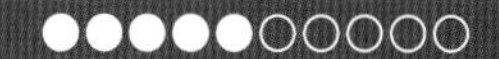

5

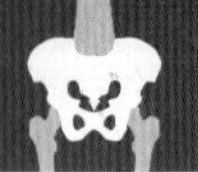

3. Orlando pelvic outcome score (1996)

Source: Cole JD, Blum DA, Ansel LJ (1996) Outcome after fixation of unstable posterior pelvic ring injuries.
Clin Orthop; (329):160–179.

Content

Type Clinician based outcome
Scale 6 subscales—4 completed by patient (12 items):

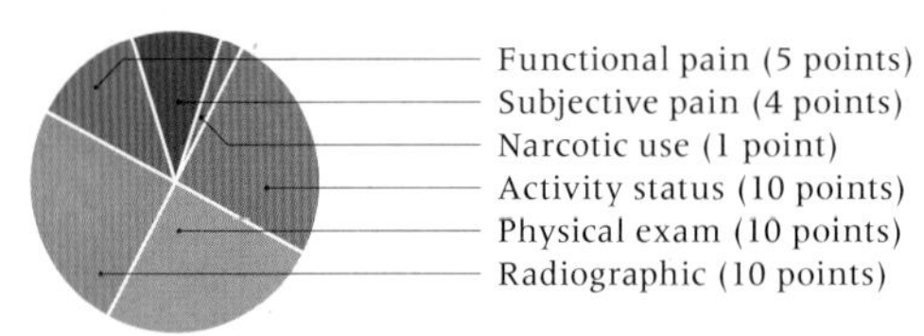

Interpretation

Minimum score: 0 points
Maximum score: 40 points

The higher the score, the higher the function.

Validation

Outcomes validated against

- SF-36

Patient population tested in	Validity	Reliability	Responsiveness
Unstable pelvic ring injuries (32 years; 56% male)	+	not tested	not tested

Validation study:
Cole JD, Blum DA, Ansel LJ (1996) Outcome after fixation of unstable posterior pelvic ring injuries. Clin Orthop; (329):160–179.

Methodological evaluation

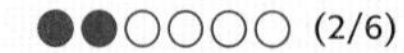
(2/6)

		no score	0 points	1 point	points
Validity	Content validity	not tested	not valid	valid	1
	Construct validity	not tested	not valid	valid	-
	Criterion validity	not tested	not valid	valid	1
Reliability	Internal consistency	not tested	not consistent	consistent	-
	Reproducibility	not tested	not reproducible	reproducible	-
	Responsiveness	not tested	not responsive	responsive	-
				Subtotal	**2**

Clinical utility

●●●○ (3/4)

	0 points	1 point	2 points	points
Patient friendliness	limited	moderate	strong	2
Clinician friendliness	limited	moderate	strong	1
			Subtotal	**3**

Total (out of 10)

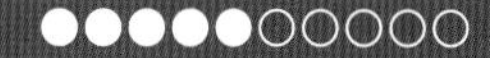

5

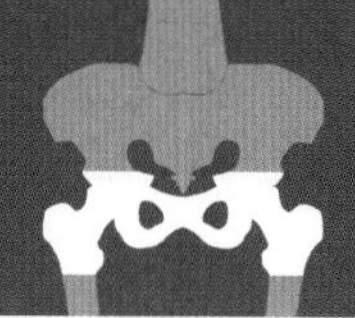

6.6 Hip

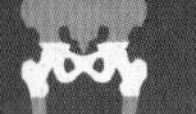

1. AAOS hip and knee score

Source: AAOS Normative Data Study and Outcomes Instruments: American Academy of Orthopaedic Surgeons
http://www.aaos.org

Content

Type Patient reported outcome
Scale 5 subscales (7 items):

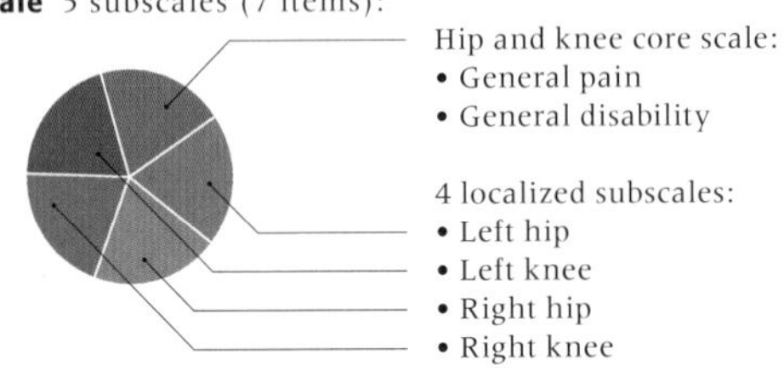

Each subscale includes 3 items to measure pain while:
- Walking on flat surfaces
- Going up or down stairs
- Lying in bed

Both a baseline and follow-up version are available.
Optional module forms for hip and knee arthroplasty patients.

Interpretation

Raw scores: mean score of all items within each category scale.

Individualized Standardized Score = 100 – [(Summed value of scale items – minimum score)/maximum score] × 100
Individual Normative Score = [(Individual score – General population mean score)/General population standard deviation] × (10 + 50)

The higher the score, the lower the function

Validation

Outcomes validated against

- WOMAC • AAOS Lower Limb Core Scale • SF-36

Patient population tested in	Validity	Reliability	Responsiveness
Patients with hip and/or knee complaints (54% male; 48 years)	+	+	+

Validation study:

Johanson NA, Liang MH, Daltroy L, et al (2004) American Academy of Orthopaedic Surgeons lower limb outcomes assessment instruments. Reliability, validity, and sensitivity to change. J Bone Joint Surg Am; 86-A: 902–909

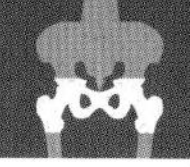

Methodological evaluation

●●●●○○ (4/6)

		no score	0 points	1 point	points
Validity	Content validity	not tested	not valid	**valid**	1
	Construct validity	not tested	not valid	**valid**	1
	Criterion validity	**not tested**	not valid	valid	-
Reliability	Internal consistency	not tested	not consistent	**consistent**	1
	Reproducibility	**not tested**	not reproducible	reproducible	-
	Responsiveness	not tested	not responsive	**responsive**	1
				Subtotal	**4**

Clinical utility

●●●● (4/4)

	0 points	1 point	2 points	points
Patient friendliness	limited	moderate	**strong**	2
Clinician friendliness	limited	moderate	**strong**	2
			Subtotal	**4**

Total (out of 10)  **8**

2. Charnley hip score (1972)

Source: Charnley J (1972) The long-term results of low-friction arthroplasty of the hip performed as a primary intervention. J Bone Joint Surg Br; 54:61–76.

Content

Type Clinician based outcome
Scale 3 subscales (18 items):

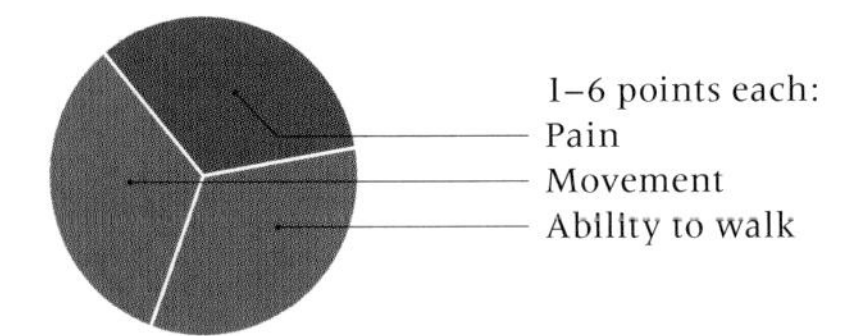

Interpretation

Each subscale graded independently.

The higher the score, the higher the function.

Validation

No validation studies were identified.

Patient population tested in	Validity	Reliability	Responsiveness
Not applicable			

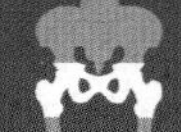

Methodological evaluation

○○○○○ (0/6)

		no score	0 points	1 point	points
Validity	Content validity	not tested	not valid	valid	-
	Construct validity	not tested	not valid	valid	-
	Criterion validity	not tested	not valid	valid	-
Reliability	Internal consistency	not tested	not consistent	consistent	-
	Reproducibility	not tested	not reproducible	reproducible	-
	Responsiveness	not tested	not responsive	responsive	-
				Subtotal	-

Clinical utility

●●●● (4/4)

	0 points	1 point	2 points	points
Patient friendliness	limited	moderate	strong	2
Clinician friendliness	limited	moderate	strong	2
			Subtotal	4

Total (out of 10) 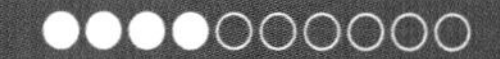 **4**

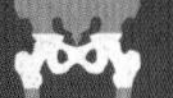

3. Functional recovery score (2000)

Source: Zuckerman JD, Koval KJ, Aharonoff GB, Hiebert R, Skovron ML (2000) A functional recovery score for elderly hip fracture patients: I. Development.
J Orthop Trauma; 14:20–25.

Content

Type Patient reported outcome
Scale 3 subscales (11 items):

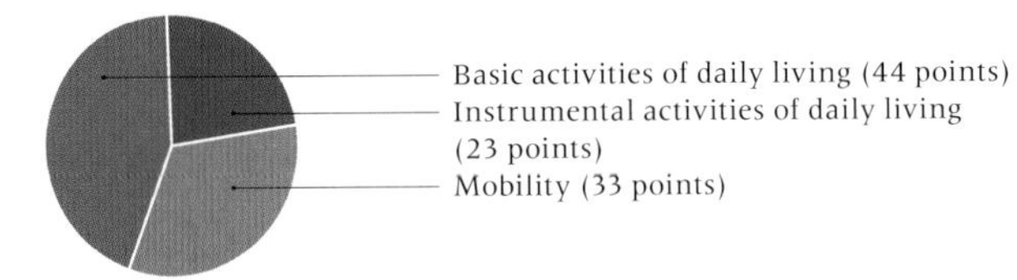

Interpretation

Minimum score: 0 points
Maximum score: 100 points

The higher the score, the higher the function.

Validation

Outcomes validated against

- Mortality
- Skilled nursing facility
- Rehospitalization

Patient population tested in	Validity	Reliability	Responsiveness
Operative treatment after proximal femur fracture (80 years; 20% male)	+	+	+

Validation study:
Zuckerman JD, Koval KJ, Aharonoff GB, et al (2000) A functional recovery score for elderly hip fracture patients: II. Validity and reliability. J Orthop Trauma; 14:26–30.

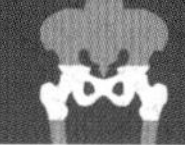

Methodological evaluation

 (5/6)

		no score	0 points	1 point	points
Validity	Content validity	not tested	not valid	**valid**	1
Validity	Construct validity	not tested	not valid	**valid**	1
Validity	Criterion validity	not tested	not valid	**valid**	1
Reliability	Internal consistency	**not tested**	not consistent	consistent	-
Reliability	Reproducibility	not tested	not reproducible	**reproducible**	1
	Responsiveness	not tested	not responsive	**responsive**	1
				Subtotal	**5**

Clinical utility

●●●● (4/4)

	0 points	1 point	2 points	points
Patient friendliness	limited	moderate	**strong**	2
Clinician friendliness	limited	moderate	**strong**	2
			Subtotal	**4**

Total (out of 10)  **9**

4. Harris hip score (1969)

Source: Harris WH (1969) Traumatic arthritis of the hip after dislocation and acetabular fractures: treatment by mold arthroplasty. An end-result study using a new method of result evaluation. J Bone Joint Surg Am; 51:737–755.

Content

Type Clinician based outcome
Scale 4 subscales (13 items):

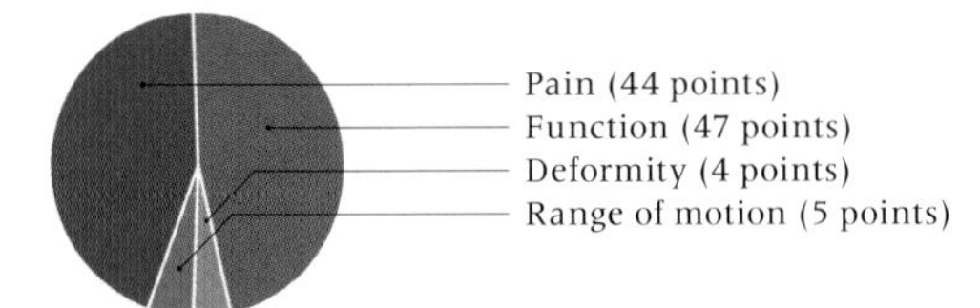

Interpretation
Excellent: 90–100 points
Good: 80–89 points
Fair: 70–79 points
Poor: < 70 points

Validation

Outcomes validated against [1]
- SF-36 [1, 2]
- WOMAC [1, 2]

Outcomes validated against [2]
- PASI [2]
- MACTAR[2]

Patient population tested in	Validity	Reliability	Responsiveness
Total hip arthroplasty (71 years; 32% male) [1]	+	+	not tested
Total hip arthroplasty (62 years; 55% male) [2]	+	not tested	+

Validation studies:

[1] Soderman P, Malchau H (2001) Is the Harris hip score system useful to study the outcome of total hip replacement? Clin Orthop; 384:189–197.
[2] Wright JG, Young N (1997) A comparison of different indices of responsiveness. J Clin Epidemiol; 50:239–246.

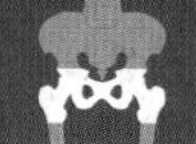

Methodological evaluation

●●●●●○ (5/6)

		no score	0 points	1 point	points
Validity	Content validity	not tested	not valid	valid	-
	Construct validity	not tested	not valid	valid	1
	Criterion validity	not tested	not valid	valid	1
Reliability	Internal consistency	not tested	not consistent	consistent	1
	Reproducibility	not tested	not reproducible	reproducible	1
	Responsiveness	not tested	not responsive	responsive	1
				Subtotal	5

Clinical utility

●●●○ (3/4)

	0 points	1 point	2 points	points
Patient friendliness	limited	moderate	strong	2
Clinician friendliness	limited	moderate	strong	1
			Subtotal	3

Total (out of 10)

●●●●●●●●○○ **8**

5. Hip disability and Osteoarthritis Outcome Score (HOOS) (2003)

Source: Nilsdotter AK, Lohmander LS, Klassbo M, Roos EM (2003) Hip disability and osteoarthritis outcome score (HOOS)--validity and responsiveness in total hip replacement.
BMC Musculoskelet Disord; 4(1):10.

Adaptation to the KOOS.

Content

Type Patient reported outcome
Scale 5 subscales (40 items):

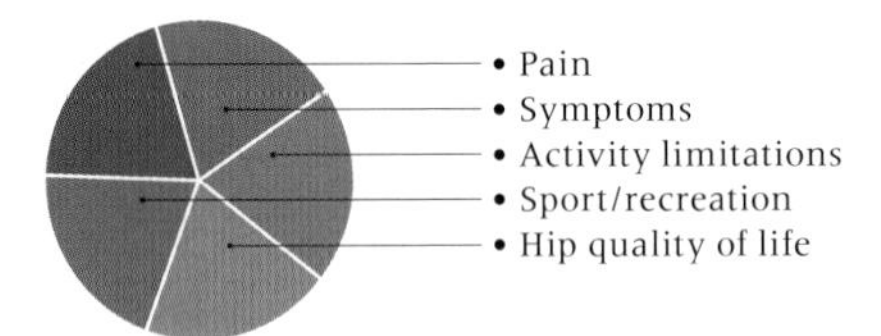

Likert scale for each item (5 choices).

WOMAC scores can be calculated from the HOOS questionnaire.

Interpretation

Scores normalized to 100 points for each subscale and each subscale scored separately.

The higher the score, the higher the function.

Validation

Outcomes validated against

- SF-36

Patient population tested in	Validity	Reliability	Responsiveness
Patients with primary hip OA evaluated for total hip replacement (71.5 years; 54% male)	+	+	+

Validation study:

Nilsdotter AK, Lohmander LS, Klassbo M, et al (2003) Hip disability and osteoarthritis outcome score (HOOS)--validity and responsiveness in total hip replacement. BMC Musculoskelet Disord; 4(1):10.

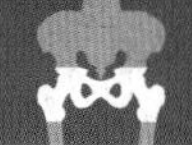

Methodological evaluation

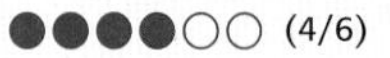 (4/6)

		no score	0 points	1 point	points
Validity	Content validity	not tested	not valid	**valid**	1
	Construct validity	not tested	not valid	**valid**	1
	Criterion validity	**not tested**	not valid	valid	-
Reliability	Internal consistency	not tested	not consistent	**consistent**	1
	Reproducibility	**not tested**	not reproducible	reproducible	-
	Responsiveness	not tested	not responsive	**responsive**	1
				Subtotal	**4**

Clinical utility

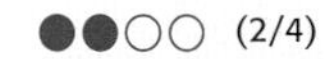 (2/4)

	0 points	1 point	2 points	points
Patient friendliness	**limited**	moderate	strong	0
Clinician friendliness	limited	moderate	**strong**	2
			Subtotal	**2**

Total (out of 10) 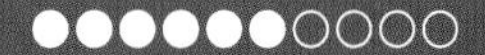 **6**

6. Hip evaluation chart 1 of Larson (1963)

Source: Larson CB (1963) Rating scale for hip disabilities. Clin Orthop; 31:85–93.

Content

Type Clinician based outcome
Scale 5 subscales (23 items):

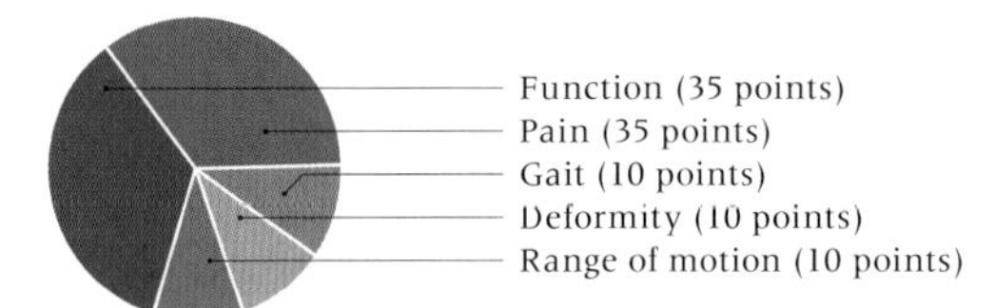

Interpretation
Minimum score: 0 points
Maximum score: 100 points

The higher the score, the higher the function.

Validation

No validation studies were identified.

Patient population tested in	Validity	Reliability	Responsiveness
Not applicable			

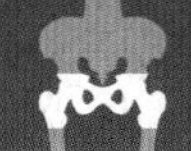

Methodological evaluation

○○○○○○ (0/6)

		no score	0 points	1 point	points
Validity	Content validity	not tested	not valid	valid	-
	Construct validity	not tested	not valid	valid	-
	Criterion validity	not tested	not valid	valid	-
Reliability	Internal consistency	not tested	not consistent	consistent	-
	Reproducibility	not tested	not reproducible	reproducible	-
	Responsiveness	not tested	not responsive	responsive	-
				Subtotal	-

Clinical utility

●●○○ (2/4)

	0 points	1 point	2 points	points
Patient friendliness	limited	moderate	strong	2
Clinician friendliness	limited	moderate	strong	0
			Subtotal	**2**

Total (out of 10) ●●○○○○○○○○ **2**

7. Hip evaluation chart 2 of Larson (1963)

Source: Larson CB (1963) Rating scale for hip disabilities. Clin Orthop; 31:85–93.

Content

Type Clinician based outcome
Scale 4 subscales (10 items):

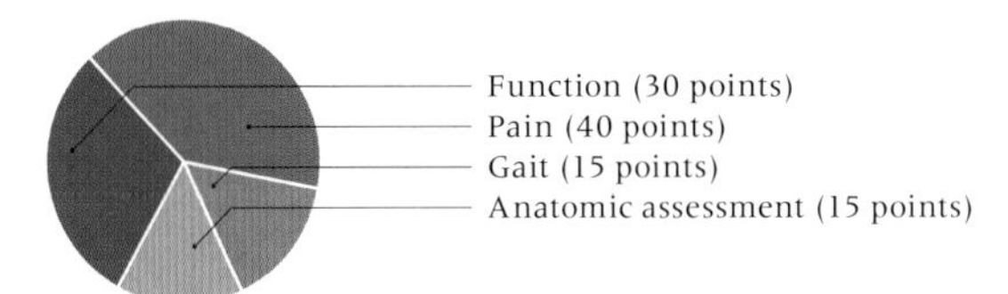

Interpretation

Minimum score: 0 points
Maximum score: 100 points

The higher the score, the higher the function.

Validation

No validation studies were identified.

Patient population tested in	Validity	Reliability	Responsiveness
Not applicable			

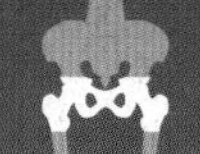

Methodological evaluation

○○○○○○ (0/6)

		no score	0 points	1 point	points
Validity	Content validity	not tested	not valid	valid	-
	Construct validity	not tested	not valid	valid	-
	Criterion validity	not tested	not valid	valid	-
Reliability	Internal consistency	not tested	not consistent	consistent	-
	Reproducibility	not tested	not reproducible	reproducible	-
	Responsiveness	not tested	not responsive	responsive	-
				Subtotal	-

Clinical utility

●●●○ (3/4)

	0 points	1 point	2 points	points
Patient friendliness	limited	moderate	strong	2
Clinician friendliness	limited	moderate	strong	1
			Subtotal	**3**

Total (out of 10) 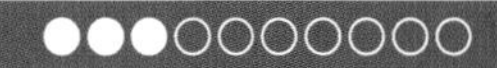 **3**

8. Hip fracture functional rating scale (1982)

Source: Keene JS, Anderson CA (1982) Hip fractures in the elderly. Discharge predictions with a functional rating scale. Jama; 248:564–567.

Content

Type Clinician based outcome
Scale 5 subscales (8 items):

Physical condition (35 points)
Ambulation (30 points)
Activities of daily living (25 points)
Prefracture living (10 points)
Disabilities (0 points—deductions)

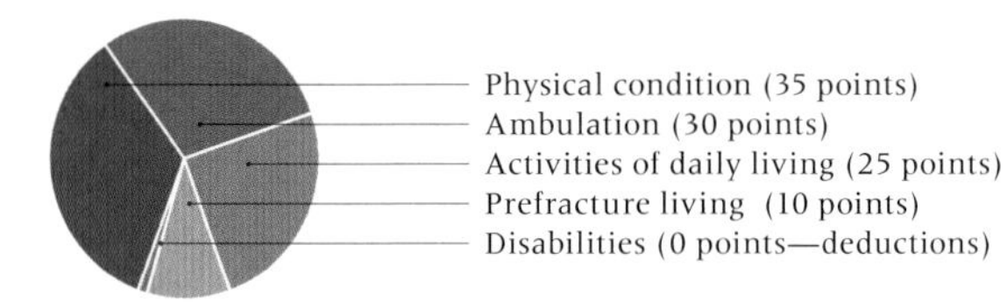

Interpretation
Minimum score: -40 points
Maximum score: 100 points

The higher the score, the lower the function.

Validation

No validation studies were identified.

Patient population tested in	Validity	Reliability	Responsiveness
Not applicable			

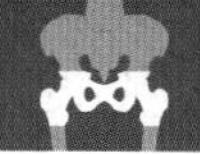

Methodological evaluation

○○○○○○ (0/6)

		no score	0 points	1 point	points
Validity	Content validity	not tested	not valid	valid	-
	Construct validity	not tested	not valid	valid	-
	Criterion validity	not tested	not valid	valid	-
Reliability	Internal consistency	not tested	not consistent	consistent	-
	Reproducibility	not tested	not reproducible	reproducible	-
	Responsiveness	not tested	not responsive	responsive	-
				Subtotal	-

Clinical utility

●●●○ (3/4)

	0 points	1 point	2 points	points
Patient friendliness	limited	moderate	strong	2
Clinician friendliness	limited	moderate	strong	1
			Subtotal	**3**

Total (out of 10) 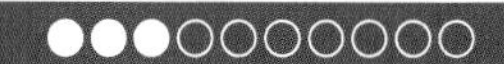 **3**

9. Hospital for Special Surgery hip score (also known as Salvati and Wilson hip score) (HSS) (1973)

Source: Salvati EA, Wilson PD Jr (1973) Long-term results of femoral-head replacement.
J Bone Joint Surg Am; 55:516–524.

Content

Type Clinician based outcome
Scale 4 subscales (24 items):

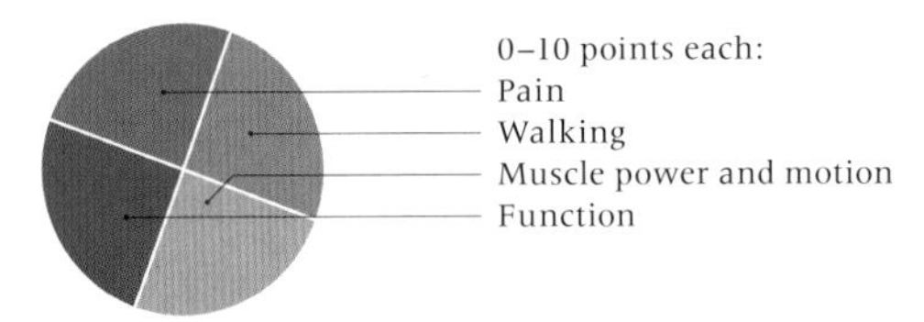

Interpretation
Excellent: ≥ 32 points
Good: 24–31 points
Fair: 16–23 points
Poor: < 16 points

Validation

No validation studies were identified.

Patient population tested in	Validity	Reliability	Responsiveness
Not applicable			

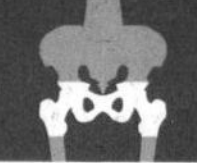

9. Hospital for Special Surgery hip score (HSS) (1973)

Methodological evaluation ○○○○○○ (0/6)

		no score	0 points	1 point	points
Validity	Content validity	not tested	not valid	valid	-
	Construct validity	not tested	not valid	valid	-
	Criterion validity	not tested	not valid	valid	-
Reliability	Internal consistency	not tested	not consistent	consistent	-
	Reproducibility	not tested	not reproducible	reproducible	-
	Responsiveness	not tested	not responsive	responsive	-
				Subtotal	-

Clinical utility ●●○○ (2/4)

	0 points	1 point	2 points	points
Patient friendliness	limited	moderate	strong	2
Clinician friendliness	limited	moderate	strong	0
			Subtotal	2

Total (out of 10) 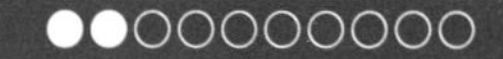 **2**

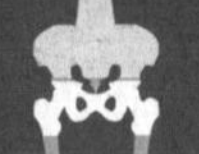

10. Lequesne - algofunctional index (1987)

Source: Lequesne MG, Mery C, Samson M, Gerard P (1987) Indexes of severity for osteoarthritis of the hip and knee. Validation--value in comparison with other assessment tests.
Scand J Rheumatol Suppl; 65:85–89.

Other versions available: German.

Content

Type Patient reported outcome
Scale 4 subscales (8 items):

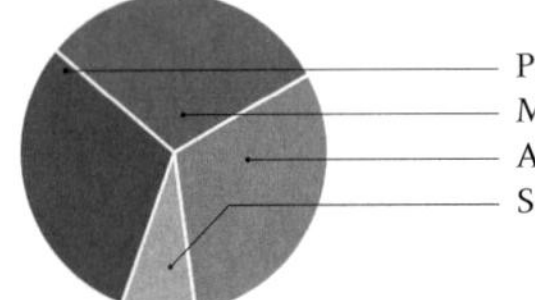

Interpretation

Minimum score: 0 points; maximum score: 26 points
The higher the score, the lower the function.

Validation

Outcomes validated against [1,2]
- Pain level, patient/physician overall opinion, walking time, and range of motion

Outcomes validated against [3]
- Radiological OA-severity and limitation in range of motion
- WOMAC

Patient population tested in	Validity	Reliability	Responsiveness
Hip osteoarthritis (age NR; sex NR) [1,2]	+	+	not tested
Hip osteoarthritis (70 years; 33% male) [3]	+/-	+/-	not tested

Validation studies:

[1] Lequesne MG, Mery C, Samson M, et al (1987) Indexes of severity for osteoarthritis of the hip and knee. Validation--value in comparison with other assessment tests. Scand J Rheumatol Suppl; 65:85–89.
[2] Lequesne MG, Samson M (1991) Indices of severity in osteoarthritis for weight bearing joints. J Rheumatol Suppl; 27:16–18.
[3] Stucki G, Sangha O, Stucki S, et al (1998) Comparison of the WOMAC (Western Ontario and McMaster Universities) osteoarthritis index and a self-report format of the self-administered Lequesne-Algofunctional index in patients with knee and hip osteoarthritis. Osteoarthritis Cartilage; 6:79–86.

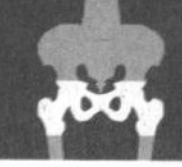

Methodological evaluation

●●○○○○ (2/6)

		no score	0 points	1 point	points
Validity	Content validity	**not tested**	not valid	valid	-
	Construct validity	not tested	**not valid**	valid	0
	Criterion validity	not tested	not valid	**valid**	1
Reliability	Internal consistency	not tested	**not consistent**	consistent	0
	Reproducibility	not tested	not reproducible	**reproducible**	1
	Responsiveness	**not tested**	not responsive	responsive	-
				Subtotal	**2**

Clinical utility

●●●○ (3/4)

	0 points	1 point	2 points	points
Patient friendliness	limited	moderate	**strong**	2
Clinician friendliness	limited	**moderate**	strong	1
			Subtotal	**3**

Total (out of 10) 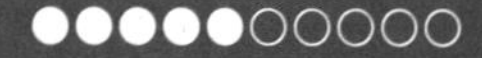 **5**

11. Lower Extremity Measure (LEM) (2000)

Source: Jaglal S, Lakhani Z, Schatzker J (2000) Reliability, validity, and responsiveness of the lower extremity measure for patients with a hip fracture.
J Bone Joint Surg Am; 82-A:955–962.

Content

Type Patient reported outcome
Scale 29 items:

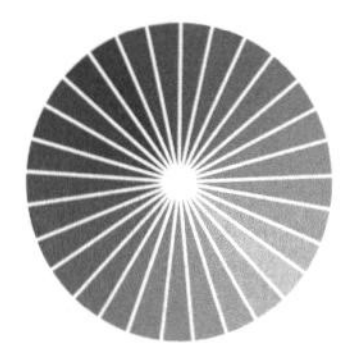

1 domain of physical disability containing 29 questions
(1–5 points or 9 points for "not applicable" for each question)

Interpretation

Scores summed and normalized to 100%.

Minimum score: 0 points
Maximum score: 100 points

The higher the score, the higher the function.

Validation

Outcomes validated against

- Timed up and go test
- SF-36
- Older Americans' resources and services

Patient population tested in	Validity	Reliability	Responsiveness
Hip fractures in the elderly (81 years; 29% male)	+	+	+

Validation study:

Jaglal S, Lakhani Z, Schatzker J (2000) Reliability, validity, and responsiveness of the lower extremity measure for patients with a hip fracture. J Bone Joint Surg Am; 82-A:955–962.

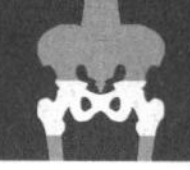

Methodological evaluation

●●●●●○ (5/6)

		no score	0 points	1 point	points
Validity	Content validity	not tested	not valid	**valid**	1
	Construct validity	not tested	not valid	**valid**	1
	Criterion validity	not tested	not valid	**valid**	1
Reliability	Internal consistency	**not tested**	not consistent	consistent	-
	Reproducibility	not tested	not reproducible	**reproducible**	1
	Responsiveness	not tested	not responsive	**responsive**	1
				Subtotal	**5**

Clinical utility

●●○○ (2/4)

	0 points	1 point	2 points	points
Patient friendliness	**limited**	moderate	strong	0
Clinician friendliness	limited	moderate	**strong**	2
			Subtotal	**2**

Total (out of 10) 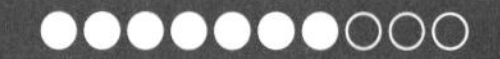 **7**

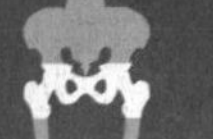

12. Mayo clinical hip score (1985)

Source: Kavanagh BF, Fitzgerald RH Jr (1985) Clinical and roentgenographic assessment of total hip arthroplasty. A new hip score.
Clin Orthop; (193):133–140.

Content

Type Clinician based outcome
Scale 2 subscales (11 items):

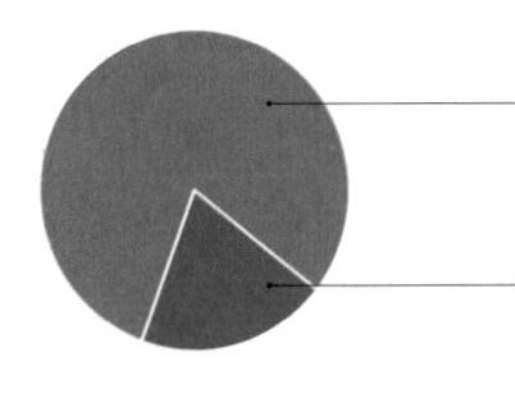

Clinical (80 points)
- Pain (40 points)
- Function (20 points)
- Mobility and power (20 points)

Radiographic (20 points)
- Acetabulum (10 points)
- Femur (10 points)

Interpretation

Excellent: 90–100 points
Good: 80–89 points
Fair: 70–79 points
Poor: < 70 points

Validation

Outcomes validated against

- Harris hip score

Patient population tested in	Validity	Reliability	Responsiveness
Revision total hip arthroplasty (age NR; sex NR)	+	not tested	not tested

Validation study:

Kavanagh BF, Fitzgerald RH Jr (1985) Clinical and roentgenographic assessment of total hip arthroplasty. A new hip score. Clin Orthop; (193): 133–140.

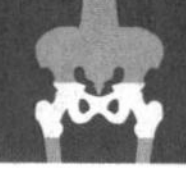

Methodological evaluation

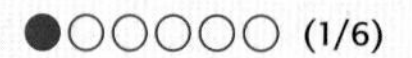 (1/6)

		no score	0 points	1 point	points
Validity	Content validity	not tested	not valid	valid	-
	Construct validity	not tested	not valid	valid	1
	Criterion validity	not tested	not valid	valid	-
Reliability	Internal consistency	not tested	not consistent	consistent	-
	Reproducibility	not tested	not reproducible	reproducible	-
	Responsiveness	not tested	not responsive	responsive	-
				Subtotal	**1**

Clinical utility

 (4/4)

	0 points	1 point	2 points	points
Patient friendliness	limited	moderate	strong	2
Clinician friendliness	limited	moderate	strong	2
			Subtotal	**4**

Total (out of 10) 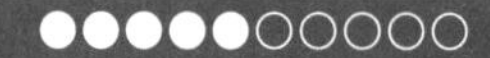 **5**

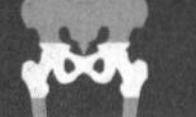

13. McMaster-Toronto Arthritis questionnaire (MACTAR) (1987)

Source: Tugwell P, Bombardier C, Buchanan WW, Goldsmith CH, Grace E, Hanna B (1987) The MACTAR Patient Preference Disability Questionnaire--an individualized functional priority approach for assessing improvement in physical disability in clinical trials in rheumatoid arthritis.
J Rheumatol; 14:446–451.

Content

Type Patient reported outcome
Scale 29 items:

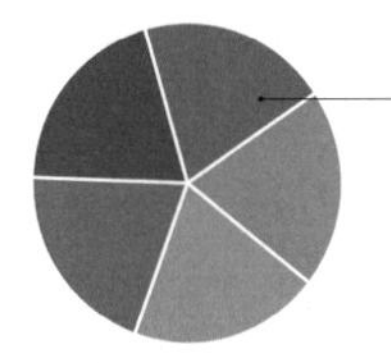

Patients identifiy and rank their 5 most important complaints preoperatively and the change (better -1 point, same 0 points, or worse +1 points) postoperatively.

Interpretation

Normalized to 100% based on initial rank and change score.
The higher the score, the higher the function.

Validation

Outcomes validated against

- WOMAC
- SF-36
- Harris hip score

Patient population tested in	Validity	Reliability	Responsiveness
Total hip arthroplasty (62 years; 55% male)	+	+	+

Validation study:

Wright JG, Young NL (1997): A comparison of different indices of responsiveness. J Clin Epidemiol; 50:239–246.

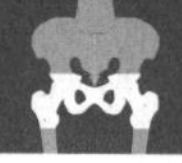

Methodological evaluation

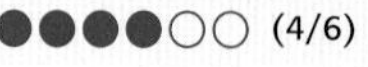 (4/6)

		no score	0 points	1 point	points
Validity	Content validity	not tested	not valid	**valid**	1
	Construct validity	not tested	not valid	**valid**	1
	Criterion validity	**not tested**	not valid	valid	-
Reliability	Internal consistency	**not tested**	not consistent	consistent	-
	Reproducibility	not tested	not reproducible	**reproducible**	1
	Responsiveness	not tested	not responsive	**responsive**	1
				Subtotal	**4**

Clinical utility

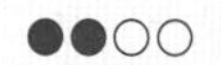 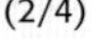 (2/4)

	0 points	1 point	2 points	points
Patient friendliness	**limited**	moderate	strong	0
Clinician friendliness	limited	moderate	**strong**	2
			Subtotal	**2**

Total (out of 10) 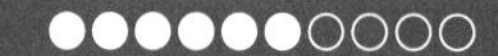 **6**

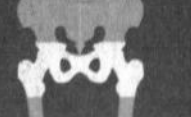

14. Merle D'Aubigne-Postel hip score (1954)

Source: D'Aubigne RM, Postel M (1954) Functional results of hip arthroplasty with acrylic prosthesis.
J Bone Joint Surg Am; 36-A(3):451–475.

Content

Type Clinician based outcome
Scale 3 subscales (18 items):

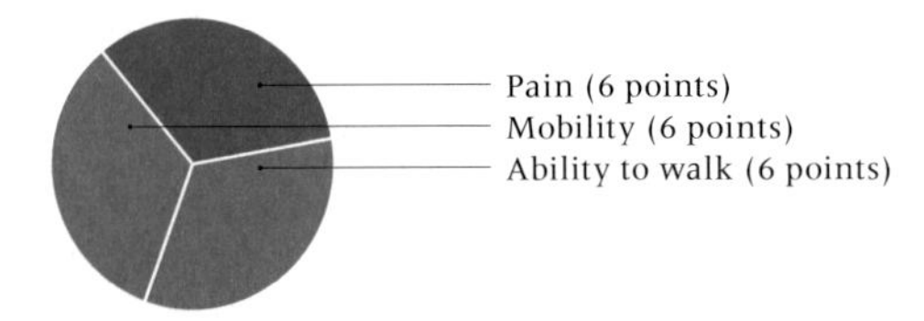

Interpretation

Excellent: 18 points
Good: 15–17 points
Fair: 12–14 points
Poor: < 12 points

Validation

No validation studies were identified.

Patient population tested in	Validity	Reliability	Responsiveness
Not applicable			

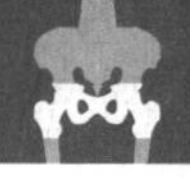

Methodological evaluation ○○○○○○ (0/6)

		no score	0 points	1 point	points
Validity	Content validity	not tested	not valid	valid	-
	Construct validity	not tested	not valid	valid	-
	Criterion validity	not tested	not valid	valid	-
Reliability	Internal consistency	not tested	not consistent	consistent	-
	Reproducibility	not tested	not reproducible	reproducible	-
	Responsiveness	not tested	not responsive	responsive	-
				Subtotal	-

Clinical utility ●●●● (4/4)

	0 points	1 point	2 points	points
Patient friendliness	limited	moderate	strong	2
Clinician friendliness	limited	moderate	strong	2
			Subtotal	**4**

Total (out of 10) ●●●●○○○○○○ **4**

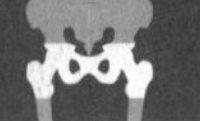

15. Non-arthritic hip score (2003)

Source: Christensen CP, Althausen PL, Mittleman MA, Lee JA, McCarthy JC (2003) The nonarthritic hip score: reliable and validated.
Clin Orthop; (406):75–83.

Content

Type Patient reported outcome
Scale 4 subscales (20 items):

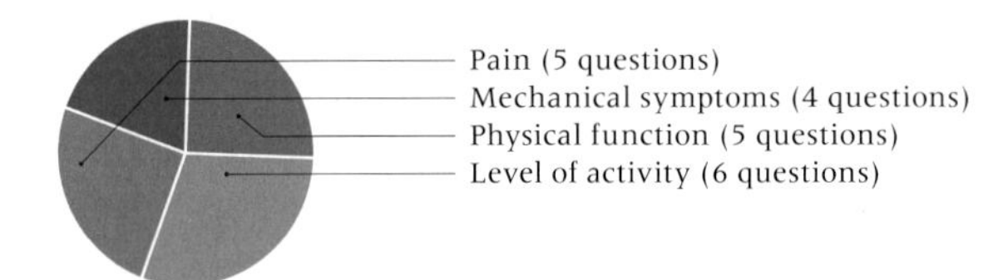

Interpretation

Minimum score: 0 points
Maximum score: 100 points

The higher the score, the higher the function.

Validation

Outcomes validated against

- Harris hip score
- SF-12

Patient population tested in	Validity	Reliability	Responsiveness
Young adults with nonarthritic hip pain (33 years; 40% male)	+	+	not tested

Validation study:
Christensen CP, Althausen PL, Mittleman MA, Lee JA, McCarthy JC (2003) The nonarthritic hip score: reliable and validated. Clin Orthop; (406): 75–83.

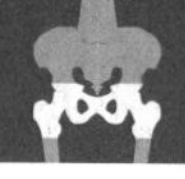

Methodological evaluation

●●●○○○ (3/6)

		no score	0 points	1 point	points
Validity	Content validity	**not tested**	not valid	valid	-
	Construct validity	not tested	not valid	**valid**	1
	Criterion validity	**not tested**	not valid	valid	-
Reliability	Internal consistency	not tested	not consistent	**consistent**	1
	Reproducibility	not tested	not reproducible	**reproducible**	1
	Responsiveness	**not tested**	not responsive	responsive	-
				Subtotal	3

Clinical utility

●●●○ (3/4)

	0 points	1 point	2 points	points
Patient friendliness	limited	**moderate**	strong	1
Clinician friendliness	limited	moderate	**strong**	2
			Subtotal	3

Total (out of 10)  **6**

16. Oxford hip score (1996)

Source: Dawson J, Fitzpatrick R, Carr A, Murray D (1996)
Questionnaire on the perceptions of patients about total hip replacement.
J Bone Joint Surg Br; 78:185–190.

Content

Type Patient reported outcome
Scale 12 items:

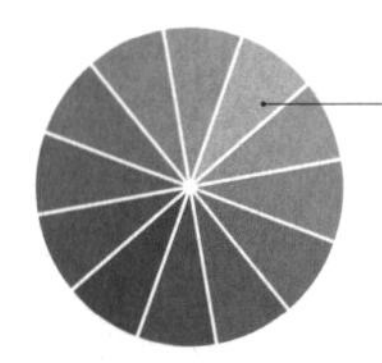

12 questions regarding perception of pain and function: 1–5 points for each

Interpretation

Minimum score: 12 points
Maximum score: 60 points
The higher the score, the lower the function.

Validation

Outcomes validated against [1]

- SF-36
- Arthritis impact measurement score
- EuroQol 5D

Outcomes validated against [2]

- EuroQol 5D

Patient population tested in	Validity	Reliability	Responsiveness
Total hip arthroplasty (71 years; 40% male) [1]	+	+	+
Revision total hip arthroplasty (68 years; 43% male) [2]	+	not tested	+

Validation studies:

[1] Dawson J, Fitzpatrick R, Carr A, et al (1996) Questionnaire on the perceptions of patients about total hip replacement. J Bone Joint Surg Br; 78:185–190.

[2] Dawson J, Fitzpatrick R, Frost S, Gundle R, McLardy-Smith P, Murray D (2001) Evidence for the validity of a patient-based instrument for assessment of outcome after revision hip replacement. J Bone Joint Surg Br; 83:1125–1129.

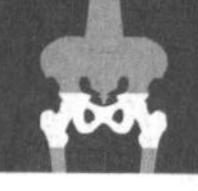

Methodological evaluation

 (5/6)

		no score	0 points	1 point	points
Validity	Content validity	not tested	not valid	valid	1
	Construct validity	not tested	not valid	valid	1
	Criterion validity	not tested	not valid	valid	-
Reliability	Internal consistency	not tested	not consistent	consistent	1
	Reproducibility	not tested	not reproducible	reproducible	1
	Responsiveness	not tested	not responsive	responsive	1
				Subtotal	**5**

Clinical utility

 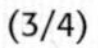 (3/4)

	0 points	1 point	2 points	points
Patient friendliness	limited	moderate	strong	1
Clinician friendliness	limited	moderate	strong	2
			Subtotal	**3**

Total (out of 10) 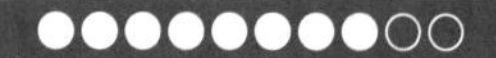 **8**

17. Parkland and Palmer mobility score (1993)

Source: Parker MJ, Palmer CR (1993) A new mobility score for predicting mortality after hip fracture.
J Bone Joint Surg Br; 75:797–798.

Content

Type Patient reported outcome
Scale 3 items:

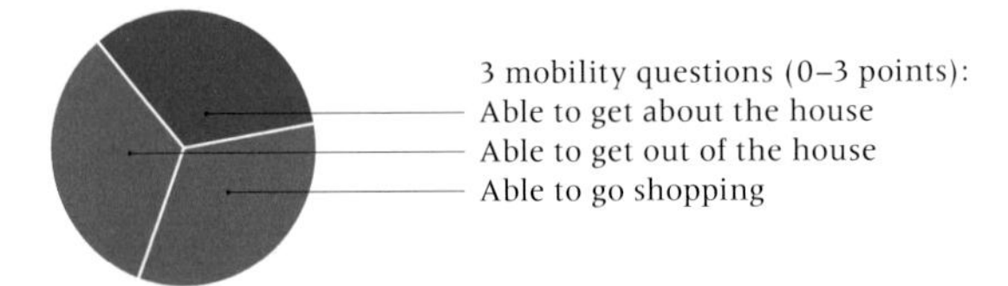

Interpretation

Minimum score: 0 points
Maximum score: 9 points

The higher the score, the higher the function.

Validation

Outcomes validated against

- Mortality at one year

Patient population tested in	Validity	Reliability	Responsiveness
Proximal femoral fracture (age NR; sex NR)	+	not tested	not tested

Validation study:
Parker MJ, Palmer CR (1993) A new mobility score for predicting mortality after hip fracture. J Bone Joint Surg Br; 75:797–798.

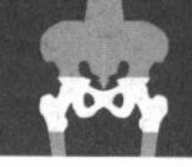

Methodological evaluation

●○○○○○ (1/6)

		no score	0 points	1 point	points
Validity	Content validity	not tested	not valid	valid	-
	Construct validity	not tested	not valid	valid	-
	Criterion validity	not tested	not valid	valid	1
Reliability	Internal consistency	not tested	not consistent	consistent	-
	Reproducibility	not tested	not reproducible	reproducible	-
	Responsiveness	not tested	not responsive	responsive	-
				Subtotal	1

Clinical utility

●●●● (4/4)

	0 points	1 point	2 points	points
Patient friendliness	limited	moderate	strong	2
Clinician friendliness	limited	moderate	strong	2
			Subtotal	4

Total (out of 10)

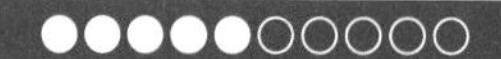

5

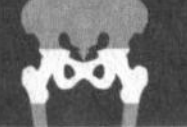

18. Patient Specific Index hip rating scale (PASI) (1994)

Source: Wright JG, Rudicel S, Feinstein AR (1994) Ask patients what they want. Evaluation of individual complaints before total hip replacement.
J Bone Joint Surg Br; 76:229–234.

Content

Type Patient reported outcome
Scale

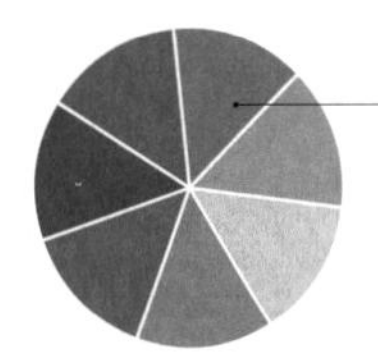

Patients rate 21 complaints for severity and importance with a 7-category ordinal scale.

Interpretation

Normalized to 100% based on total sum of importance-severity scores divided by maximum possible score.

Minimum score: 0 points
Maximum score: 100 points

The higher the score, the lower the function.

Validation

Outcomes validated against

- WOMAC
- SF-36
- Harris hip score

Patient population tested in	Validity	Reliability	Responsiveness
Total hip arthroplasty (62 years; 55% male)	+	+	+

Validation study:
Wright JG, Young N (1997): A comparison of different indices of responsiveness. J Clin Epidemiol; 50:239–246.

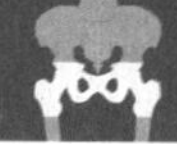

Methodological evaluation

●●●●○○ (4/6)

		no score	0 points	1 point	points
Validity	Content validity	not tested	not valid	valid	1
	Construct validity	not tested	not valid	valid	1
	Criterion validity	not tested	not valid	valid	-
Reliability	Internal consistency	not tested	not consistent	consistent	-
	Reproducibility	not tested	not reproducible	reproducible	1
	Responsiveness	not tested	not responsive	responsive	1
				Subtotal	**4**

Clinical utility

●●○○ (2/4)

	0 points	1 point	2 points	points
Patient friendliness	limited	moderate	strong	0
Clinician friendliness	limited	moderate	strong	2
			Subtotal	**2**

Total (out of 10)  **6**

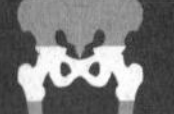

19. Rheumatoid and Arthritis Outcome Score for the lower extremtiy (RAOS) (2003)

Source: Bremander AB, Petersson IF, Roos EM (2004) Validation of the Rheumatoid and Arthritis Outcome Score (RAOS) for the lower extremity. Health Qual Life Outcomes; 1(1):55.

Adaptation to the KOOS.

Content

Type Patient reported outcome
Scale 5 subscales (42 items):

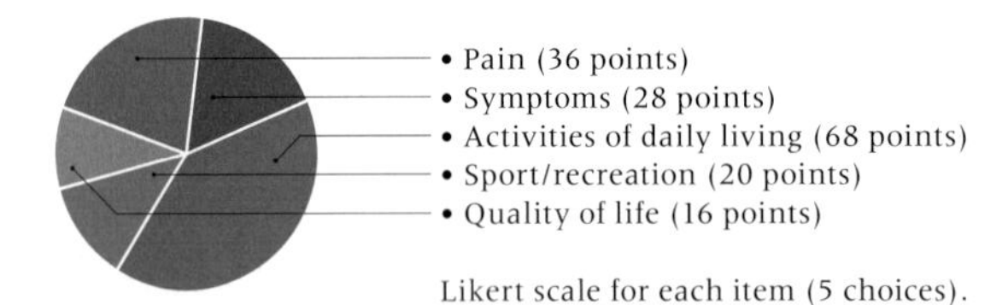

Likert scale for each item (5 choices).

Interpretation

Scores normalized to 100 points for each subscale and each subscale scored separately.

The higher the score, the higher the function.

Validation

Outcomes validated against

- Health assessment questionnaire
- SF-36
- Arthritis impact measurement scale

Patient population tested in	Validity	Reliability	Responsiveness
Patients with chronic inflammatory joint disease (56 years; 27% male)	+	+	+

Validation study:

Source: Bremander AB, Petersson IF, Roos EM (2004) Validation of the Rheumatoid and Arthritis Outcome Score (RAOS) for the lower extremity. Health Qual Life Outcomes; 1(1):55.

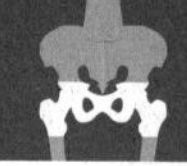

Methodological evaluation

●●●●●○ (5/6)

		no score	0 points	1 point	points
Validity	Content validity	not tested	not valid	valid	1
	Construct validity	not tested	not valid	valid	1
	Criterion validity	not tested	not valid	valid	-
Reliability	Internal consistency	not tested	not consistent	consistent	1
	Reproducibility	not tested	not reproducible	reproducible	1
	Responsiveness	not tested	not responsive	responsive	1
				Subtotal	**5**

Clinical utility

●●○○ (2/4)

	0 points	1 point	2 points	points
Patient friendliness	limited	moderate	strong	0
Clinician friendliness	limited	moderate	strong	2
			Subtotal	**2**

Total (out of 10) 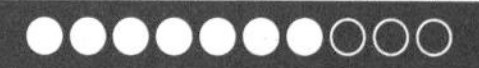 **7**

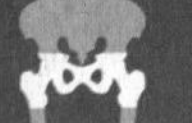

20. Thompson and Epstein score (1951)

Source: Thompson VP, Epstein HC (1951) Traumatic dislocation of the hip; a survey of two hundred and four cases covering a period of twenty-one years.
J Bone Joint Surg Am; 33-A(3):746–778.

Content

Type Clinician based outcome
Scale 2 subscales (6 items):

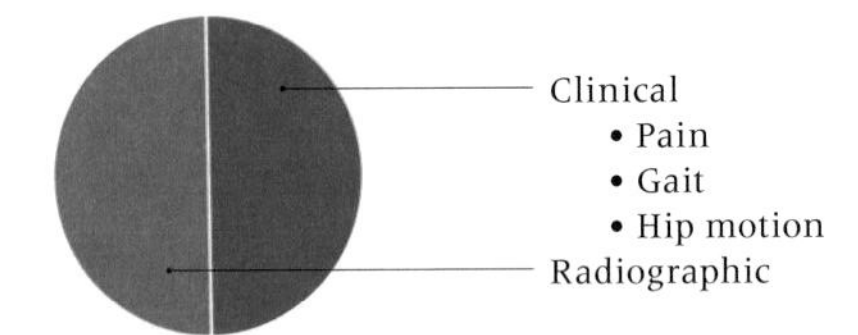

Interpretation

Clinical and radiographic:
Excellent
Good
Fair
Poor
(no points – based on qualitative findings)

Validation

No validation studies were identified.

Patient population tested in	Validity	Reliability	Responsiveness
Not applicable			

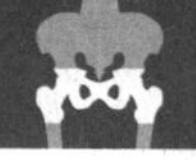

Methodological evaluation

○○○○○○ (0/6)

		no score	0 points	1 point	points
Validity	Content validity	not tested	not valid	valid	-
	Construct validity	not tested	not valid	valid	-
	Criterion validity	not tested	not valid	valid	-
Reliability	Internal consistency	not tested	not consistent	consistent	-
	Reproducibility	not tested	not reproducible	reproducible	-
	Responsiveness	not tested	not responsive	responsive	-
				Subtotal	-

Clinical utility

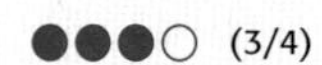

(3/4)

	0 points	1 point	2 points	points
Patient friendliness	limited	moderate	strong	2
Clinician friendliness	limited	moderate	strong	1
			Subtotal	3

Total (out of 10)

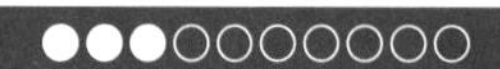

3

21. Total hip arthroplasty outcome evaluation (1991)

Source: Liang MH, Katz JN, Phillips C, Sledge C, Cats-Baril W (1991) The total hip arthroplasty outcome evaluation form of the American Academy of Orthopaedic Surgeons. Results of a nominal group process. The American Academy of Orthopaedic Surgeons Task Force on Outcome Studies.
J Bone Joint Surg Am; 73:639–646.

Content

Type Patient reported outcome
Scale 5 subscales (5 items):

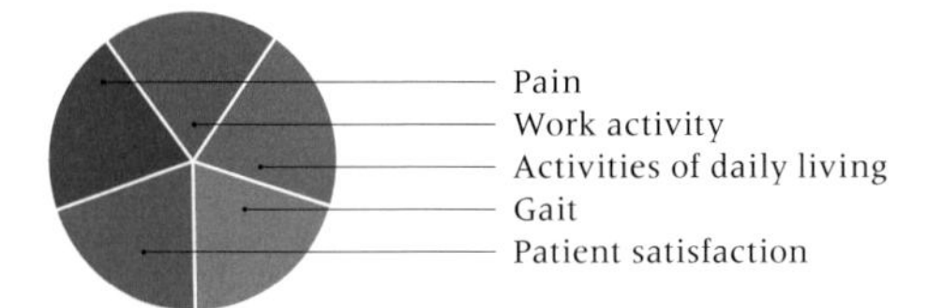

Interpretation

Minimum score: 0 points
Maximum score: 100 points

Scoring or interpretation not specified.

Validation

Outcomes validated against

- Sickness impact profile

Patient population tested in	Validity	Reliability	Responsiveness
Total hip arthroplasty (60 years; 33% male)	+	+	not tested

Validation study:
Katz JN, Phillips CB, Poss R,et al (1995) The validity and reliability of a Total Hip Arthroplasty Outcome Evaluation Questionnaire. J Bone Joint Surg Am; 77:1528–1534.

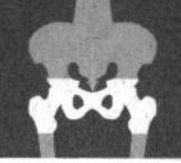

Methodological evaluation

●●○○○○ (2/6)

		no score	0 points	1 point	points
Validity	Content validity	not tested	not valid	valid	-
	Construct validity	not tested	not valid	valid	1
	Criterion validity	not tested	not valid	valid	-
Reliability	Internal consistency	not tested	not consistent	consistent	-
	Reproducibility	not tested	not reproducible	reproducible	1
	Responsiveness	not tested	not responsive	responsive	-
				Subtotal	**2**

Clinical utility

●●○○ (2/4)

	0 points	1 point	2 points	points
Patient friendliness	limited	moderate	strong	2
Clinician friendliness	limited	moderate	strong	0
			Subtotal	**2**

Total (out of 10) 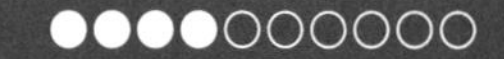 **4**

22. Western Ontario and McMaster Universities OA index (WOMAC) (1988)

Source: Bellamy N, Buchanan WW, Goldsmith CH, Campbell J, Stitt LW (1988) Validation study of WOMAC: a health status instrument for measuring clinically important patient relevant outcomes to antirheumatic drug therapy in patients with osteoarthritis of the hip or knee. J Rheumatol; 15:1833–1840.

Other versions available: Swedish, German.

Content

Type Patient reported outcome
Scale 3 subscales (41 items):

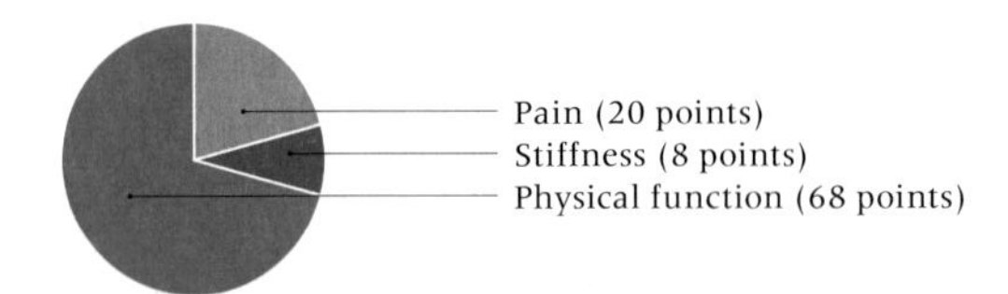

Interpretation

Minimum score: 0 points
Maximum score: 96 points

The higher the score, the lower the function.

Validation

Outcomes validated against [1, 5]

- SF-36

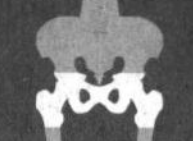

Validation (cont)

Patient population tested in	Validity	Reliability	Responsiveness
Total hip arthroplasty (71 years; 34% male) [1,2]	+	+	not tested
Total hip arthroplasty (62 years; 55% male) [3]	not tested	+	+
Hip osteoarthritis (70 years; 33% male) [4]	+	+	not tested
Hip osteoarthritis (55 years; 20% male) [5]	+	+	not tested

Validation studies:

[1] Soderman P, Malchau H (2001) Is the Harris hip score system useful to study the outcome of total hip replacement? Clin Orthop; 384:189–197.

[2] Soderman P, Malchau H: (2000) Validity and reliability of Swedish WOMAC osteoarthritis index: a self-administered disease-specific questionnaire (WOMAC) versus generic instruments (SF-36 and NHP). Acta Orthop Scand; 71:39–46.

[3] Wright JG, Young N (1997): A comparison of different indices of responsiveness. J Clin Epidemiol; 50:239–246.

[4] Stucki G, Sangha O, Stucki S, et al (1998) Comparison of the WOMAC (Western Ontario and McMaster Universities) osteoarthritis index and a self-report format of the self-administered Lequesne Algofunctional index in patients with knee and hip osteoarthritis. Osteoarthritis Cartilage; 6:79–86.

[5] Thumboo J, Chew LH, Soh CH (2001) Validation of the Western Ontario and Mcmaster University osteoarthritis index in Asians with osteoarthritis in Singapore. Osteoarthritis Cartilage; 9:440–446.

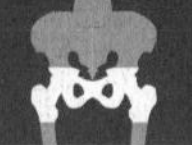

22. Western Ontario and McMaster Universities OA index (WOMAC) (1988)

Details see previous pages.

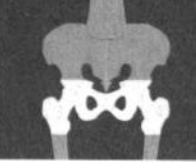

Methodological evaluation

●●●●●● (6/6)

		no score	0 points	1 point	points
Validity	Content validity	not tested	not valid	valid	1
	Construct validity	not tested	not valid	valid	1
	Criterion validity	not tested	not valid	valid	1
Reliability	Internal consistency	not tested	not consistent	consistent	1
	Reproducibility	not tested	not reproducible	reproducible	1
	Responsiveness	not tested	not responsive	responsive	1
				Subtotal	6

Clinical utility

●●●○ (3/4)

	0 points	1 point	2 points	points
Patient friendliness	limited	moderate	strong	1
Clinician friendliness	limited	moderate	strong	2
			Subtotal	3

Total (out of 10) 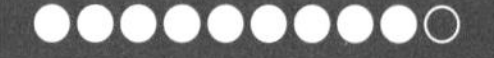 **9**

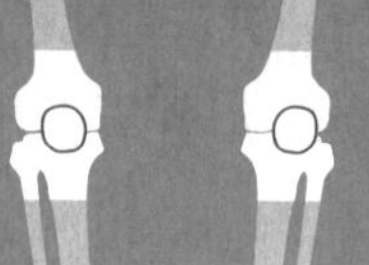

6.7 Knee

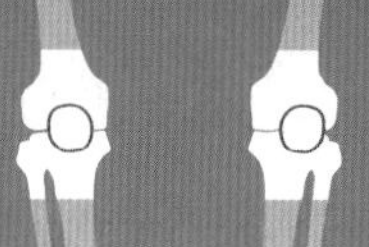

1. AAOS hip and knee score

Source: AAOS Normative Data Study and Outcomes Instruments: American Academy of Orthopaedic Surgeons
http://www.aaos.org

Content

Type Patient reported outcome
Scale 5 subscales (7 items):

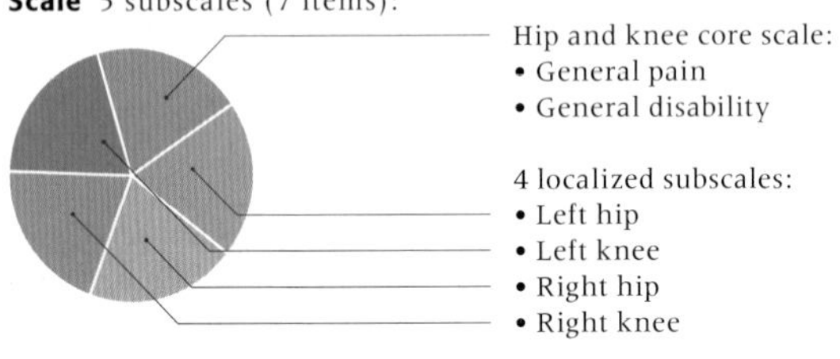

Each subscale includes 3 items to measure pain while:
- Walking on flat surfaces
- Going up or down stairs
- Lying in bed

Both a baseline and follow-up version are available.
Optional module forms for hip and knee arthroplasty patients.

Interpretation

Raw scores: mean score of all items within each category scale.

Individualized Standardized score = 100 – [(Summed value of scale items – minimum score)/maximum score] × 100
Individual Normative Score = [(Individual score – General population mean score)/General population standard deviation] × (10 + 50)

The higher the score, the lower the function.

Validation

Outcomes validated against

- WOMAC
- AAOS lower limb core scale
- SF-36

Patient population tested in	Validity	Reliability	Responsiveness
Patients with hip and/or knee complaints (54% male; 48 years)	+	+	+

Validation study:

Johanson NA, Liang MH, Daltroy L, et al (2004) American Academy of Orthopaedic Surgeons lower limb outcomes assessment instruments. Reliability, validity, and sensitivity to change. J Bone Joint Surg Am; 86-A: 902–909.

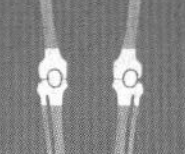

Methodological evaluation

●●●●○○ (4/6)

		no score	0 points	1 point	points
Validity	Content validity	not tested	not valid	**valid**	1
	Construct validity	not tested	not valid	**valid**	1
	Criterion validity	**not tested**	not valid	valid	-
Reliability	Internal consistency	not tested	not consistent	**consistent**	1
	Reproducibility	not tested	not reproducible	**reproducible**	1
	Responsiveness	**not tested**	not responsive	responsive	-
				Subtotal	**4**

Clinical utility

●●●● (4/4)

	0 points	1 point	2 points	points
Patient friendliness	limited	moderate	**strong**	2
Clinician friendliness	limited	moderate	**strong**	2
			Subtotal	**4**

Total (out of 10) 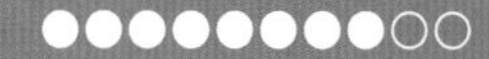 **8**

2. AAOS sports knee scale

Source: AAOS Normative Data Study and Outcomes Instruments:
American Academy of Orthopaedic Surgeons
http://www.aaos.org

Content

Type Patient reported outcome
Scale 6 subscales (27 items):

Sports knee core (7 items)
Knee catch (4 items)
Knee lock (4 items)
Pre injury activity limitation (4 items)
Current activity limitation (4 items)
Pain on activity (4 items)

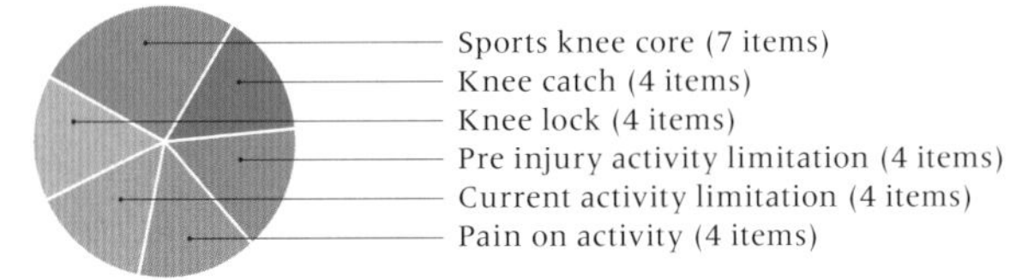

Global scale that can be used alone with focus on lower limb as a whole or with the hip/knee or ankle/foot module.

Interpretation

Raw scores: mean score of all items within each category scale.

Individualized Standardized score = 100 – [(Summed value of scale items – minimum score)/maximum score] × 100
Individual Normative Score = [(Individual score – General population mean score)/General population standard deviation] × (10 + 50)

The higher the score, the lower the function.

Validation

Outcomes validated against

- WOMAC
- SF-36
- Physician assessment

Patient population tested in	Validity	Reliability	Responsiveness
Patients with hip and/or knee complaints (54% male; 48 years)	+	+	+

Validation study:

Johanson NA, Liang MH, Daltroy L, et al (2004) American Academy of Orthopaedic Surgeons lower limb outcomes assessment instruments. Reliability, validity, and sensitivity to change. J Bone Joint Surg Am; 86-A: 902–909.

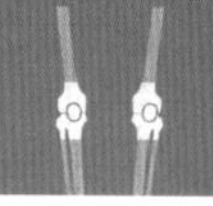

Methodological evaluation

●●●●○○ (4/6)

		no score	0 points	1 point	points
Validity	Content validity	not tested	not valid	valid	1
	Construct validity	not tested	not valid	valid	1
	Criterion validity	not tested	not valid	valid	-
Reliability	Internal consistency	not tested	not consistent	consistent	1
	Reproducibility	not tested	not reproducible	reproducible	1
	Responsiveness	not tested	not responsive	responsive	-
				Subtotal	**4**

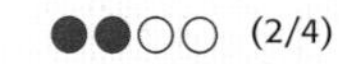

Clinical utility

●●○○ (2/4)

	0 points	1 point	2 points	points
Patient friendliness	limited	moderate	strong	0
Clinician friendliness	limited	moderate	strong	2
			Subtotal	**2**

Total (out of 10) ●●●●●●○○○○ **6**

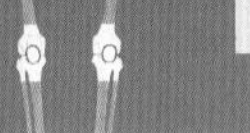

3. ACL evaluation format (1987)

Source: Lukianov AV, Gillquist J, Grana WA and DeHaven KE (1987) An anterior cruciate ligament (ACL) evaluation format for assessment of artificial or autologous anterior cruciate reconstruction results. Clin Orthop; 167–180.

Content

Type Clinician based outcome
Scale 3 subscales (38 items):

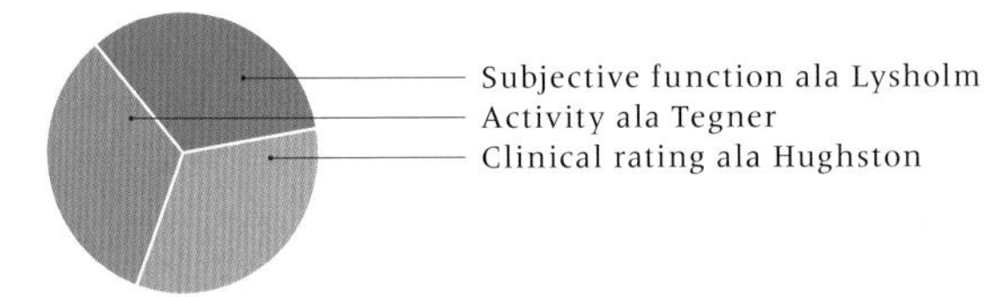

Interpretation

Not a rating scale, rather a data collection system.

Validation

No validation studies were identified.

Patient population tested in	Validity	Reliability	Responsiveness
Not applicable			

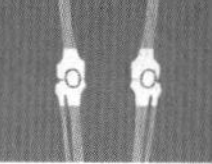

Methodological evaluation 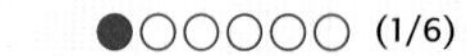 (1/6)

		no score	0 points	1 point	points
Validity	Content validity	not tested	not valid	**valid**	1
	Construct validity	**not tested**	not valid	valid	-
	Criterion validity	**not tested**	not valid	valid	-
Reliability	Internal consistency	**not tested**	not consistent	consistent	-
	Reproducibility	**not tested**	not reproducible	reproducible	-
	Responsiveness	**not tested**	not responsive	responsive	-
				Subtotal	**1**

Clinical utility 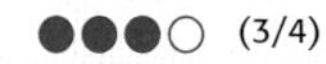 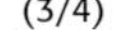 (3/4)

	0 points	1 point	2 points	points
Patient friendliness	limited	moderate	**strong**	2
Clinician friendliness	limited	**moderate**	strong	1
			Subtotal	**3**

Total (out of 10) 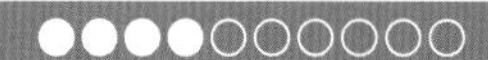 **4**

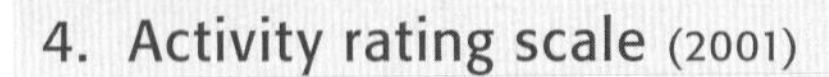

4. Activity rating scale (2001)

Source: Marx RG, Stump TJ, Jones EC, Wickiewicz TL, Warren RF (2001) Development and evaluation of an activity rating scale for disorders of the knee.
Am J Sports Med; 29:213–218.

Content

Type Patient reported outcome
Scale 4 subscales (4 items):

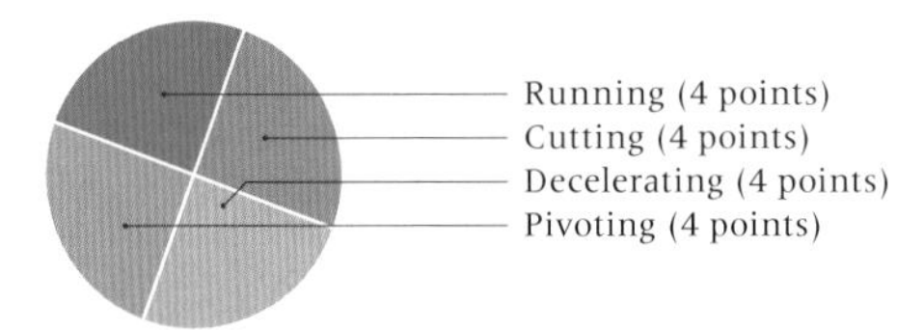

Interpretation

Minimum: 0 points
Maximum: 16 points

The higher the score, the higher the activity.

Validation

Outcomes validated against

- Tegner activity level rating scale
- Cincinnati knee rating system
- Daniel scale

Patient population tested in	Validity	Reliability	Responsiveness
Healthy volunteers (34 years; 68% male)	+	+	not tested

Validation study:

Marx RG, Stump TJ, Jones EC, et al (2001) Development and evaluation of an activity rating scale for disorders of the knee. Am J Sports Med; 29:213–218.

Methodological evaluation

●●●●○○ (4/6)

		no score	0 points	1 point	points
Validity	Content validity	not tested	not valid	valid	1
	Construct validity	not tested	not valid	valid	1
	Criterion validity	not tested	not valid	valid	1
Reliability	Internal consistency	not tested	not consistent	consistent	-
	Reproducibility	not tested	not reproducible	reproducible	1
	Responsiveness	not tested	not responsive	responsive	-
				Subtotal	**4**

Clinical utility

 (4/4)

	0 points	1 point	2 points	points
Patient friendliness	limited	moderate	strong	2
Clinician friendliness	limited	moderate	strong	2
			Subtotal	**4**

Total (out of 10) 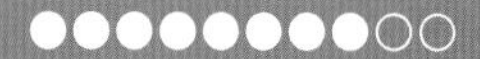 **8**

5. American Knee Society score (AKS) (1989)

Source: Insall JN, Dorr LD, Scott RD, Scott WN (1989) Rationale of the Knee Society clinical rating system.
Clin Orthop; (248):13–14.

Content

Type Clinician based outcome
Scale 7 subscales (10 items):

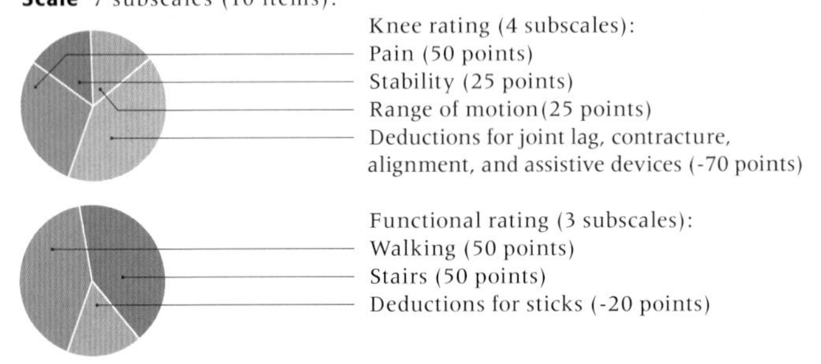

Interpretation

Knee rating:
Minimum score: 0 points; maximum score: 100 points
The higher the score, the higher the function.
Functional rating:
Minimum score: 0 points; maximum score: 100 points
The higher the score, the higher the function.

Validation

Outcomes validated against

- SF-36
- WOMAC

Patient population tested in	Validity	Reliability	Responsiveness
TKA (70 years; 41% male) [1]	+	not tested	-
TKA (70 years; 37% male) [2]	not tested	+	not tested
TKA (age NR; sex NR) [3]	not tested	+	not tested

Validation studies:

[1] Lingard EA, Katz JN, Wright RJ, et al (2001) Validity an responsiveness of the Knee Society Clinical Rating System in comparison with the SF-36 and WOMAC. J Bone Joint Surg Am; 83-A:1856–1964.
[2] Bach CM, Nogler M, Steingruber IE, et al (2002) Scoring systems in total knee arthroplasty. Clin Orthop; (399):184–196.
[3] Liow RY, Walker K, Wajid MA, et al (2003) Functional rating for knee arthroplasty: comparison of three scoring systems. Orthopedics; 26: 143–149.

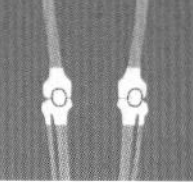

Methodological evaluation

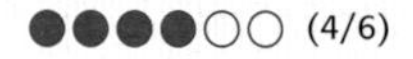 (4/6)

		no score	0 points	1 point	points
Validity	Content validity	not tested	not valid	valid	1
	Construct validity	not tested	not valid	valid	1
	Criterion validity	not tested	not valid	valid	1
Reliability	Internal consistency	not tested	not consistent	consistent	-
	Reproducibility	not tested	not reproducible	reproducible	1
	Responsiveness	not tested	not responsive	responsive	0
				Subtotal	**4**

Clinical utility

●●●○ (3/4)

	0 points	1 point	2 points	points
Patient friendliness	limited	moderate	strong	2
Clinician friendliness	limited	moderate	strong	1
			Subtotal	**3**

Total (out of 10)  **7**

6. Bristol (1988)

Source: Mackinnon J, Young S and Baily RA (1988) The St Georg sledge for unicompartmental replacement of the knee. A prospective study of 115 cases.
J Bone Joint Surg Br; 70:217–223.

Content

Type Clinician based outcome
Scale 4 subscales (9 items):

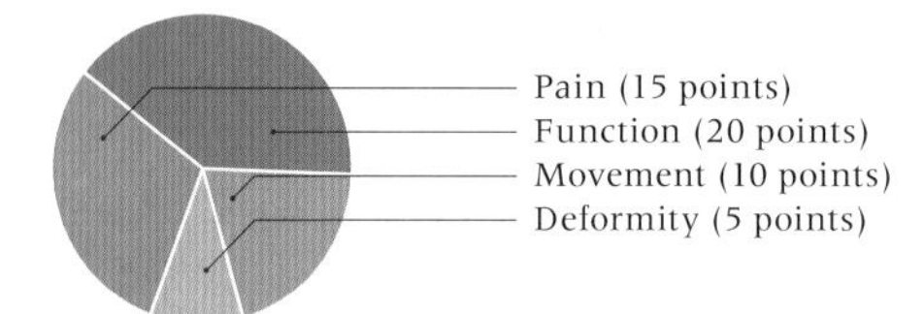

Interpretation

Excellent: 41–50 points
Good: 36–40 points
Fair: 30–35 points
Poor: < 30 points

Validation

No validation studies were identified.

Patient population tested in	Validity	Reliability	Responsiveness
Total knee arthroplasty (70 years; 37% male)	not tested	+	not tested

Validation study:
Bach CM, Nogler M, Steingruber IE, Ogon M, Wimmer C, Gobel G and Krismer M (2002)Scoring systems in total knee arthroplasty. Clin Orthop; (399):184–196.

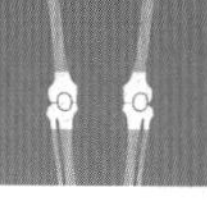

Methodological evaluation

●○○○○○ (1/6)

		no score	0 points	1 point	points
Validity	Content validity	not tested	not valid	valid	-
	Construct validity	not tested	not valid	valid	-
	Criterion validity	not tested	not valid	valid	-
Reliability	Internal consistency	not tested	not consistent	consistent	-
	Reproducibility	not tested	not reproducible	reproducible	1
	Responsiveness	not tested	not responsive	responsive	-
				Subtotal	**1**

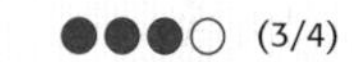

Clinical utility

●●●○ (3/4)

	0 points	1 point	2 points	points
Patient friendliness	limited	moderate	strong	2
Clinician friendliness	limited	moderate	strong	1
			Subtotal	**3**

Total (out of 10) ●●●●○○○○○○ **4**

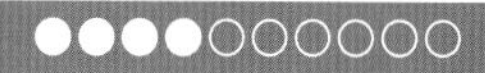

7. British Orthopaedic Association knee functional assessment chart (1978)

Source: Aichroth P, Freeman MAR, Smillie IS and Souter WA (1987) A knee function assessment chart. From the British Orthopaedic Association Research Sub-Committee.
J Bone Joint Surg Br; 60-B:308–309.

Content

Type Clinician based outcome
Scale 2 subscales (12 items):

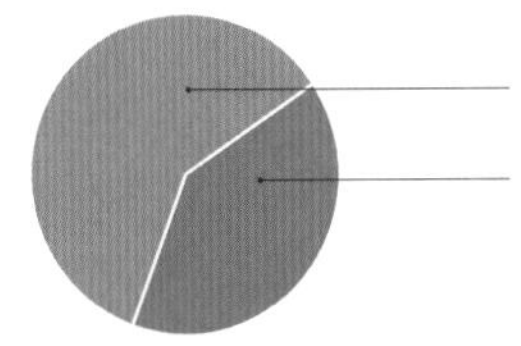

Interpretation

Minimum score: 11 points
Maximum score: 55 points

The higher the score, the higher the function.

Validation

No validation studies were identified.

Patient population tested in	Validity	Reliability	Responsiveness
Total knee arthroplasty (age NR; sex NR)	not tested	+	not tested

Validation study:
Liow RY, Walker K, Wajid MA, Bedi G and Lennox CM: Functional rating for knee arthroplasty: comparison of three scoring systems. Orthopedics; 26:143–149.

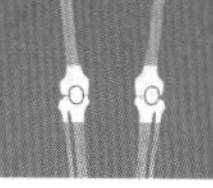

Methodological evaluation 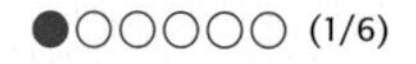 (1/6)

		no score	0 points	1 point	points
Validity	Content validity	not tested	not valid	valid	-
	Construct validity	not tested	not valid	valid	-
	Criterion validity	not tested	not valid	valid	-
Reliability	Internal consistency	not tested	not consistent	consistent	-
	Reproducibility	not tested	not reproducible	reproducible	1
	Responsiveness	not tested	not responsive	responsive	-
				Subtotal	**1**

Clinical utility ●●●● (4/4)

	0 points	1 point	2 points	points
Patient friendliness	limited	moderate	strong	2
Clinician friendliness	limited	moderate	strong	2
			Subtotal	**4**

Total (out of 10) 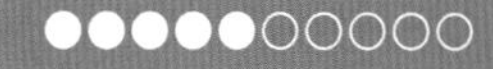 **5**

8. Cincinnati knee rating system (1983)

Sources: Noyes FR, Mooar PA, Matthews DS and Butler DL (1983) The symptomatic anterior cruciate-deficient knee. Part I: the long-term functional disability in athletically active individuals. J Bone Joint Surg Am; 65:154–162.
Noyes FR, Barber SD and Mooar LA (1989) A rationale for assessing sports activity levels and limitations in knee disorders. Clin Orthop: (246):238–249.
Noyes FR, Barber SD and Mangine RE (1990) Bone-patellar ligament-bone and fascia lata allografts for reconstruction of the anterior cruciate ligament. J Bone Joint Surg Am; 72:1125–1136.

Content

Type Clinician based outcome
Scale 6 subscales (28 items—8 completed by patient):

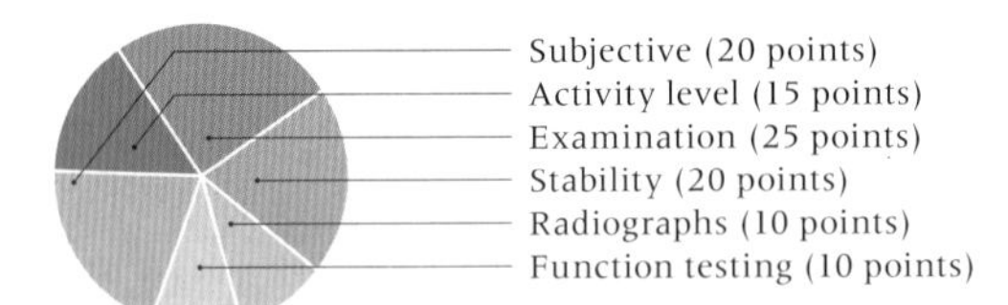

Interpretation

Excellent: All subscales grade excellent (may have 1 in good)
Good: All subscales grade excellent or good
Fair: Any one subscale grading fair
Poor: Any one subscale grading poor

Validation

Outcomes validated against [1]

- HSS
- Lysholm knee function scoring scale

Outcomes validated against [2]

- SF-36
- ADL
- AAOS sports knee scale
- Patient rating
- Clinician rating

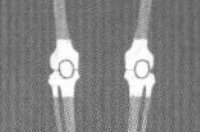

Validation (cont)

Patient population tested in	Validity	Reliability	Responsiveness
Anterior cruciate ligament surgery (25 years; sex NR) [1]	+	not tested	+
Athlete with variety of knee disorders (32 years; 52% male) [2]	not tested	+	+
Anterior cruciate ligament surgery (28 years; 53% male) [3]	not tested	not tested	+
Chronic knee pain (36 years; 56% male) [4]	not tested	+	not tested
Normal knee (34 years; 44% male) [4]	not tested	+	not tested

Validation studies:

[1] Sgaglione NA, Del Pizzo W, Fox JM, et al (1995) Critical analysis of knee ligament rating systems. Am J Sports Med; 23:660-667.

[2] Marx RG, Jones EC, Allen AA, et al (2001) Reliability, validity, and responsiveness of four knee outcome scales for athletic patients. J Bone Joint Surg Am; 83-A:1459-1469.

[3] Risberg MA, Holm I, Steen H, et al (1999) Sensitivity to changes over time for the IKDC form, the Lysholm score, and the Cincinnati knee score. A prospective study of 120 ACL reconstructed patients with a 2-year follow-up. Knee Surg Sports Traumatol Arthrosc; 7:152-159.

[4] Barber-Westin SD, Noyes FR, et al (1999) Rigorous statistical reliability, validity, and responsiveness testing of the Cincinnati knee rating system in 350 subjects with uninjured, injured, or anterior cruciate ligament-reconstructed knees. Am J Sports Med; 27:402-416.

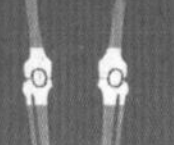

8. Cincinnati knee rating system (1983)

Details see previous pages.

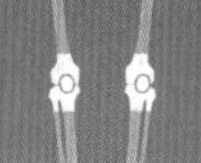

Methodological evaluation

 (5/6)

		no score	0 points	1 point	points
Validity	Content validity	not tested	not valid	valid	1
	Construct validity	not tested	not valid	valid	1
	Criterion validity	not tested	not valid	valid	1
Reliability	Internal consistency	not tested	not consistent	consistent	-
	Reproducibility	not tested	not reproducible	reproducible	1
	Responsiveness	not tested	not responsive	responsive	1
				Subtotal	**5**

Clinical utility

●●○○ (2/4)

	0 points	1 point	2 points	points
Patient friendliness	limited	moderate	strong	2
Clinician friendliness	limited	moderate	strong	0
			Subtotal	**2**

Total (out of 10)  **7**

9. Fulkerson-Shea patellofemoral joint evaluation score (1990)

Source: Fulkerson JP, Shea KP (1990) Disorders of patellofemoral alignment.
J Bone Joint Surg Am; 72:1424–1429.

Content

Type Clinician based outcome
Scale 7 subscales (7 items):

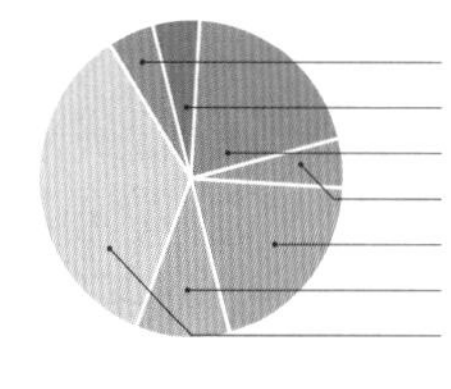

Interpretation

Excellent: 91–100 points
Good: 81–90 points
Fair: 70–80 points
Poor: < 70 points

Validation

Outcomes validated against

- Lysholm knee function scoring scale
- KPS
- MFA
- SF-36
- Tegner activity level rating scale

Patient population tested in	Validity	Reliability	Responsiveness
Patients with acute patellar dislocation (46% male; 16 years)	+	not tested	not tested
Patients with acute patellar dislocation (41% male; 16 years)	not tested	+	not tested

Validation study:

Paxton EW, Fithian DC, Stone ML, et al (2003) The reliability and validity of knee-specific and general health instruments in assessing acute patellar dislocation outcomes. Am J Sports Med; 31:487–492.

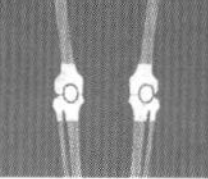

Methodological evaluation

●●●●○○ (4/6)

		no score	0 points	1 point	points
Validity	Content validity	not tested	not valid	valid	1
	Construct validity	not tested	not valid	valid	1
	Criterion validity	not tested	not valid	valid	1
Reliability	Internal consistency	not tested	not consistent	consistent	-
	Reproducibility	not tested	not reproducible	reproducible	1
	Responsiveness	not tested	not responsive	responsive	-
				Subtotal	**4**

Clinical utility

●●●● (4/4)

	0 points	1 point	2 points	points
Patient friendliness	limited	moderate	strong	2
Clinician friendliness	limited	moderate	strong	2
			Subtotal	**4**

Total (out of 10)  **8**

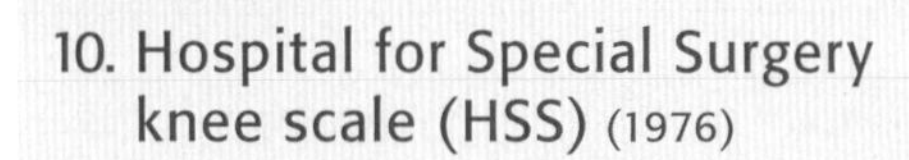

10. Hospital for Special Surgery knee scale (HSS) (1976)

Source: Ranawat CS, Insall J, Shine J (1976) Duo-condylar knee arthroplasty: hospital for special surgery design. Clin Orthop; 00(120):76-82.

Content

Type Clinician based outcome
Scale 6 subscales (7 items):

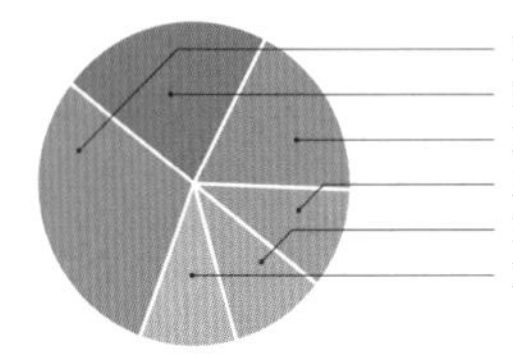

Interpretation

Excellent: 85–100 points
Good: 70–84 points
Fair: 60–69 points
Poor < 60 points

Validation

Outcomes validated against [1]

- Lysholm knee function scoring scale
- Cincinnati knee rating system

Outcomes validated against [2]

- Several objective and subjective measures

Patient population tested in	Validity	Reliability	Responsiveness
Anterior cruciate ligament surgery (25 years; sex NR) [1]	+	not tested	not tested
Total knee arthroplasty (63 years; 100% male) [2]	+	not tested	not tested
Total knee arthroplasty (70 years; 37% male) [3]	not tested	+	not tested

Validation studies:

[1] Sgaglione NA, Del Pizzo W, Fox JM, et al (1995) Critical analysis of knee ligament rating systems. Am J Sports Med; 23:660–667.
[2] Gore DR, Murray MP, Sepic SB, et al (1986) Correlations between objective measures of function and a clinical knee rating scale following total knee replacement. Orthopedics; 9:1363–1367.
[3] Bach CM, Nogler M, Steingruber IE, et al (2002) Scoring systems in total knee arthroplasty. Clin Orthop; (399):184–196.

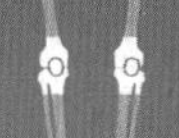

Methodological evaluation

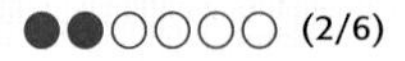 (2/6)

		no score	0 points	1 point	points
Validity	Content validity	not tested	not valid	valid	-
	Construct validity	not tested	not valid	valid	-
	Criterion validity	not tested	not valid	valid	1
Reliability	Internal consistency	not tested	not consistent	consistent	-
	Reproducibility	not tested	not reproducible	reproducible	1
	Responsiveness	not tested	not responsive	responsive	-
				Subtotal	**2**

Clinical utility

●●●○ (3/4)

	0 points	1 point	2 points	points
Patient friendliness	limited	moderate	strong	2
Clinician friendliness	limited	moderate	strong	1
			Subtotal	**3**

Total (out of 10) 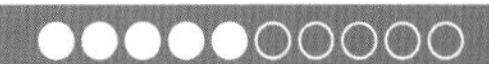 **5**

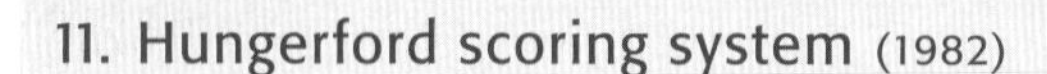

11. Hungerford scoring system (1982)

Source: Hungerford DS, Kenna RV, Krackow KA (1982)
The porous-coated anatomic total knee.
Orthop Clin North Am; 13:103–122.

Content

Type Clinician based outcome
Scale 5 subscales (6 items):

Pain (40 points)
Stability (10–20 points)
Deformity (15 to -20 points)
Mobility (25 points)
Quadriceps strength (10 points)

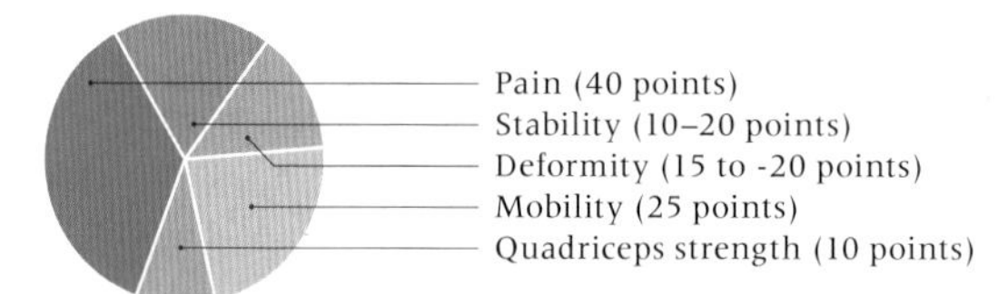

Interpretation

Minimum score: -20 points
Maximum score: 100 points

The higher the score, the higher the function.

Validation

No validation studies were identified.

Patient population tested in	Validity	Reliability	Responsiveness
Total knee arthroplasty (70 years; 37% male)	not tested	+	not tested

Validation study:

Bach CM, Nogler M, Steingruber IE, et al (2002) Scoring systems in total knee arthroplasty. Clin Orthop; (399):184–196.

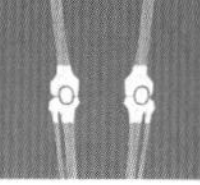

Methodological evaluation

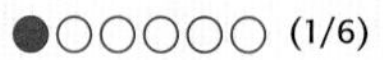 (1/6)

		no score	0 points	1 point	points
Validity	Content validity	not tested	not valid	valid	-
	Construct validity	not tested	not valid	valid	-
	Criterion validity	not tested	not valid	valid	-
Reliability	Internal consistency	not tested	not consistent	consistent	-
	Reproducibility	not tested	not reproducible	reproducible	1
	Responsiveness	not tested	not responsive	responsive	-
				Subtotal	**1**

Clinical utility

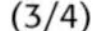 (3/4)

	0 points	1 point	2 points	points
Patient friendliness	limited	moderate	strong	2
Clinician friendliness	limited	moderate	strong	1
			Subtotal	**3**

Total (out of 10) 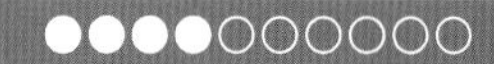 **4**

12. International Knee Documentation Committee knee scoring system (IKDC)

(2001)

Source: Irrgang JJ, Anderson AF, Boland AL, Harner CD, Kurosaka M, Neyret P, Richmond JC, Shelborne KD (2001) Development and validation of the international knee documentation committee subjective knee form.
Am J Sports Med; 29:600–613.

Content

Type Patient reported outcome
Scale 3 subscales (45 items):

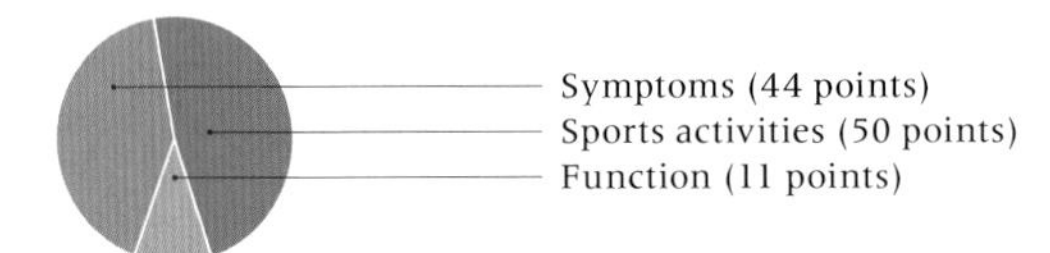

Interpretation

Scores summed and normalized to 100.
Minimum score: 0 points; maximum score: 100 points
The higher the score, the higher the function.

Validation

Outcomes validated against [1]
- SF-36
- Cincinnati knee rating system

Outcomes validated against [2]
- Cincinnati knee rating system
- VAS, range of motion
- KT-1000

Patient population tested in	Validity	Reliability	Responsiveness
Variety of knee injuries (38 years; 53% male) [1]	+	not tested	not tested
Variety of knee injuries (37 years; 61% male) [1]	not tested	+	not tested
Anterior cruciate ligament reconstruction (28 years; 53% male) [2]	+	not tested	-

Validation studies:

[1] Irrgang JJ, Anderson AF, Boland AL, et al (2001) Development and validation of the international knee documentation committee subjective knee form. Am J Sports Med; 29:600–613.
[2] Risberg MA, Holm I, Steen H, et al (1999) Sensitivity to changes over time for the IKDC form, the Lysholm score, and the Cincinnati knee score. A prospective study of 120 ACL reconstructed patients with a 2-year follow-up. Knee Surg Sports Traumatol Arthrosc; 7:152–159.

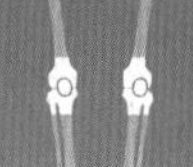

Methodological evaluation

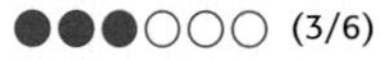 (3/6)

		no score	0 points	1 point	points
Validity	Content validity	not tested	not valid	valid	-
	Construct validity	not tested	not valid	valid	1
	Criterion validity	not tested	not valid	valid	1
Reliability	Internal consistency	not tested	not consistent	consistent	-
	Reproducibility	not tested	not reproducible	reproducible	1
	Responsiveness	not tested	not responsive	responsive	0
				Subtotal	**3**

Clinical utility

●●○○ (2/4)

	0 points	1 point	2 points	points
Patient friendliness	limited	moderate	strong	0
Clinician friendliness	limited	moderate	strong	2
			Subtotal	**2**

Total (out of 10) 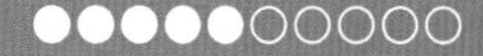 **5**

13. Iowa knee evaluation (1989)

Source: Merchant TC, Dietz FR (1989) Long-term follow-up after fractures of the tibial and fibular shafts.
J Bone Joint Surg Am; 71:599–606.

Content

Type Clinician based outcome
Scale 5 subscales (18 items):

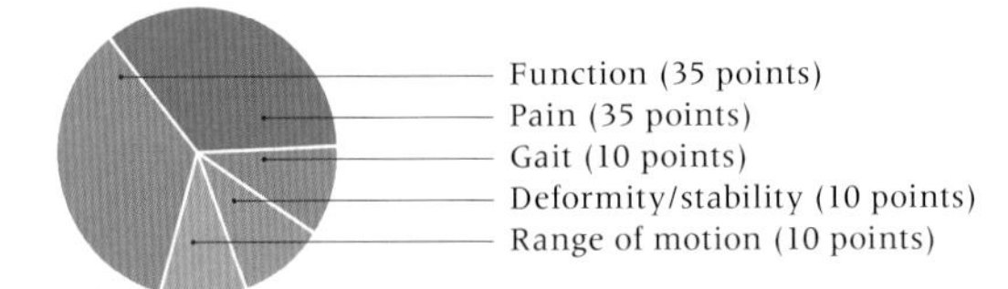

Interpretation

Excellent: 90–100 points
Good: 80–89 points
Fair: 70–79 points
Poor: < 70 points

Validation

No validation studies were identified.

Patient population tested in	Validity	Reliability	Responsiveness
Not applicable			

Methodological evaluation

○○○○○○ (0/6)

		no score	0 points	1 point	points
Validity	Content validity	not tested	not valid	valid	-
	Construct validity	not tested	not valid	valid	-
	Criterion validity	not tested	not valid	valid	-
Reliability	Internal consistency	not tested	not consistent	consistent	-
	Reproducibility	not tested	not reproducible	reproducible	-
	Responsiveness	not tested	not responsive	responsive	-
				Subtotal	-

Clinical utility

●●●○ (3/4)

	0 points	1 point	2 points	points
Patient friendliness	limited	moderate	strong	2
Clinician friendliness	limited	moderate	strong	1
			Subtotal	**3**

Total (out of 10) 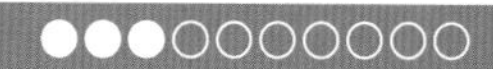 **3**

15. Knee outcome survey activities of daily living scale (1998)

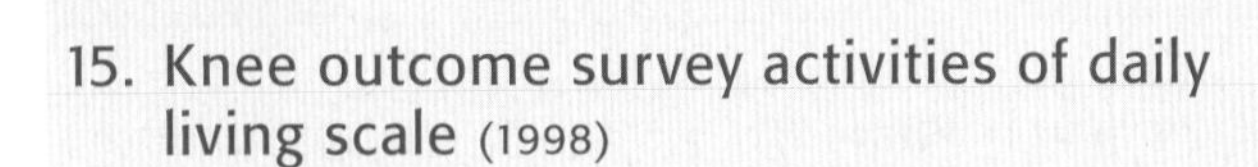

Source: Irrgang JJ, Snyder-Mackler L, Fu FH (1998) Development of a patient-reported measure of function of the knee. JBJS; 8A:1132–1145.

Content

Type Patient reported outcome
Scale 2 subscales (10 items):

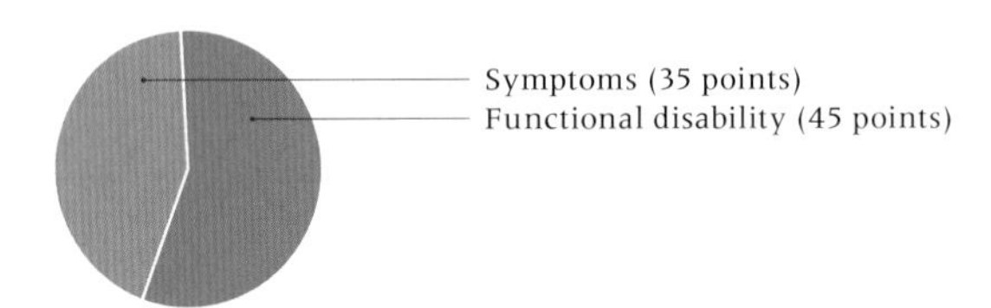

Interpretation
Minimum score: 0 points; maximum score: 80 points
The higher the score, the higher the function.

Validation

Outcomes validated against [1]
- SF-36
- Cincinnati knee rating system
- Lysholm knee function scoring scale
- AAOS sports knee scale
- Patient rating
- Clinician rating

Outcomes validated against [2]
- Lysholm knee function scoring scale
- Global rating

Patient population tested in	Validity	Reliability	Responsiveness
Athlete with variety of knee disorders (32 years; 52% male) [1]	+	+	not tested
Variety of operative and nonoperative knee disorders (33 years; 58% male) [2]	+	+	+

Validation studies:

[1] Marx RG, Jones EC, Allen AA, et al (2001) Reliability, validity, and responsiveness of four knee outcome scales for athletic patients. J Bone Joint Surg Am; 83-A:1459–1469.

[2] Irrgang JJ, Snyder-Mackler L, Fu FH (1998) Development of a patient-reported measure of function of the knee. JBJS; 8A:1132–1145.

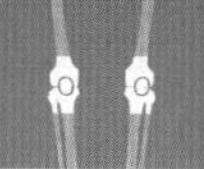

Methodological evaluation

●●●●●● (6/6)

		no score	0 points	1 point	points
Validity	Content validity	not tested	not valid	valid	1
	Construct validity	not tested	not valid	valid	1
	Criterion validity	not tested	not valid	valid	1
Reliability	Internal consistency	not tested	not consistent	consistent	1
	Reproducibility	not tested	not reproducible	reproducible	1
	Responsiveness	not tested	not responsive	responsive	1
				Subtotal	**6**

Clinical utility

●●●● (4/4)

	0 points	1 point	2 points	points
Patient friendliness	limited	moderate	strong	2
Clinician friendliness	limited	moderate	strong	2
			Subtotal	**4**

Total (out of 10) ○○○○○○○○○○ **10**

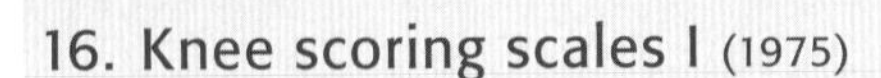

16. Knee scoring scales I (1975)

Source: Kettelkamp DB, Thompson C (1975) Development of a knee scoring scale.
Clin Orthop; (107):93–109.

Content

Type Clinician based outcome
Scale 2 subscales (13 items):

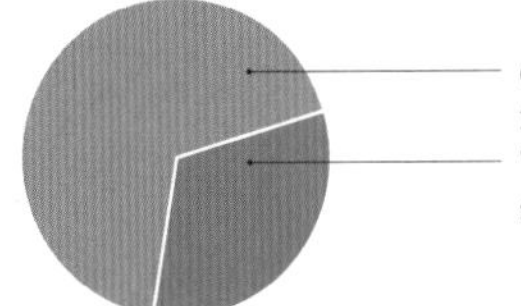

6 items regarding perception of pain and function (70 points)
7 items regarding knee motion, stability and deformity (33 points)

Interpretation

Minimum score: 0 points
Maximum score: 103 points

The higher the score, the higher the function.

Validation

Outcomes validated against

- Knee motion during stance phase of gait

Patient population tested in	Validity	Reliability	Responsiveness
Meniscectomy, OA, and RA (age NR; sex NR)	+	not tested	not tested

Validation study:

Kettelkamp DB, Thompson C (1975) Development of a knee scoring scale. Clin Orthop; (107):93–109.

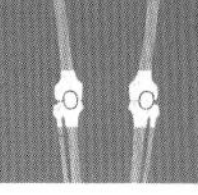

Methodological evaluation

●○○○○○ (1/6)

		no score	0 points	1 point	points
Validity	Content validity	not tested	not valid	valid	-
	Construct validity	not tested	not valid	valid	-
	Criterion validity	not tested	not valid	valid	1
Reliability	Internal consistency	not tested	not consistent	consistent	-
	Reproducibility	not tested	not reproducible	reproducible	-
	Responsiveness	not tested	not responsive	responsive	-
				Subtotal	**1**

Clinical utility

●●●● (4/4)

	0 points	1 point	2 points	points
Patient friendliness	limited	moderate	strong	2
Clinician friendliness	limited	moderate	strong	2
			Subtotal	**4**

Total (out of 10) ●●●●●○○○○○ **5**

14. Knee injury and Osteoarthritis Outcome Score (KOOS) (1998)

Source: Roos EM, Roos HP, Lohmander LS, Ekdahl C and Beynnon BD (1998) Knee Injury and Osteoarthritis Outcome Score (KOOS)--development of a self-administered outcome measure. J Orthop Sports Phys Ther; 28:88–96.

Content

Type Patient reported outcome
Scale 5 subscales (42 items):

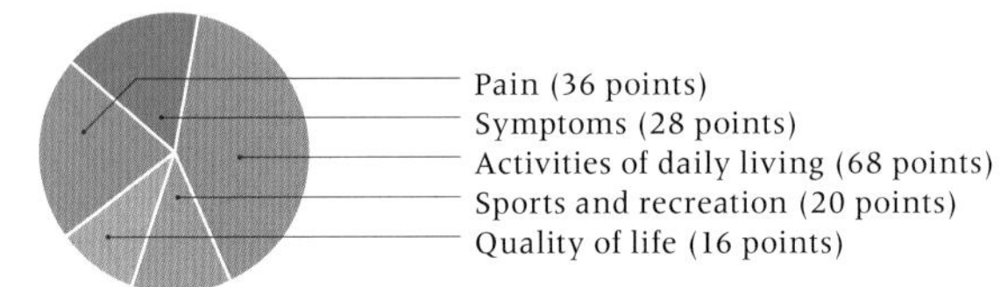

Interpretation

Scores normalized to 100 points for each subscale and each subscale scored separately.
Minimum subscale score: 0 points
Maximum subscale score: 100 points
The higher the score, the higher the function.

Validation

Outcomes validated against [1]
- SF-36

Outcomes validated against [2]
- SF-36
- Lysholm knee function scoring scale

Patient population tested in	Validity	Reliability	Responsiveness
Anterior cruciate ligament injury (32 years; 43% male) [1]	+	not tested	+
Anterior cruciate ligament injury (age NR; sex NR) [1]	not tested	+	not tested
Variety of preoperative knee injuries (40 years; 37% male) [2]	+	+	+

Validation studies:

[1] Roos EM, Roos HP, Lohmander LS, et al (1989) Knee Injury and Osteoarthritis Outcome Score (KOOS)--development of a self-administered outcome measure. J Orthop Sports Phys Ther; 28:88–96.

[2] Roos EM, Roos HP, Ekdahl C, et al (1998) Knee injury and Osteoarthritis Outcome Score (KOOS)--validation of a Swedish version. Scand J Med Sci Sports; 8:439–448.

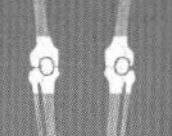

Methodological evaluation

●●●●●● (6/6)

		no score	0 points	1 point	points
Validity	Content validity	not tested	not valid	valid	1
	Construct validity	not tested	not valid	valid	1
	Criterion validity	not tested	not valid	valid	1
Reliability	Internal consistency	not tested	not consistent	consistent	1
	Reproducibility	not tested	not reproducible	reproducible	1
	Responsiveness	not tested	not responsive	responsive	1
				Subtotal	**6**

Clinical utility

●●○○ (2/4)

	0 points	1 point	2 points	points
Patient friendliness	limited	moderate	strong	0
Clinician friendliness	limited	moderate	strong	2
			Subtotal	**2**

Total (out of 10) ●●●●●●●●○○ **8**

17. Kujala Patellofemoral Score (also know as the AKPS–Anterior Knee Pain Scale) (1993)

Source: Kujala UM, Jaakkola LH, Koskinen SK, Taimela S, Nelimarkka O (1993) Scoring of patellofemoral disorders. Arthroscopy; 9:159–163.

Content

Type Clinician based outcome
Scale 13 items evaluating subjective symptons and fuctional limitations:

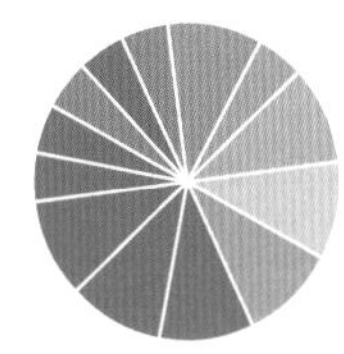

Limp (5 points)
Support (5 points)
Walking (5 points)
Stairs (10 points)
Squatting (5 points)
Running (10 points)
Jumping (10 points)
Prolonged sitting with knees flexed (10 points)
Pain (10 points)
Swelling (10 points)
Subluxations (10 points)
Atrophy of thigh (5 points)
Flexion deficiency (5 points)

Interpretation
Minimum score: 0 points
Maximum score: 100 points

The higher the score, the higher the function.

Validation

Outcomes validated against [1]
- Lateral patellar tilt and displacement with quad extension (MRI)
- Increasing levels of patellofemoral disability

Outcomes validated against [2]
- Visual analog scales for activity related pain

Outcomes validated against [3]
- KDC
- Lysholm
- MFA
- SF-36
- Fulkerson
- Tegner

Validation (cont)

Patient population tested in	Validity	Reliability	Responsiveness
All females with: no pain (28.6 years) anterior knee pain (28.5 years) subluxation (23.9 years) dislocation (23.8 years) [1]	+	not tested	not tested
Patients with patellofemoral pain (35% male; 12–40 years) [2]	+	+	+
Patients with acute patellar dislocation and prior subluxation/dislocation (46% male; 16 years) [3]	+	not tested	not tested
Patients with acute patellar dislocation and prior subluxation/dislocation (41% male; 16 years) [3]	not tested	+	not tested

Validation studies:

[1] Kujala UM, Jaakkola LH, Koskinen SK, et al (1993) Scoring of patellofemoral disorders. Arthroscopy; 9:159–163.

[2] Crossley KM, Bennell KL, Cowan SM et al (2004) Analysis of outcome measures for persons with patellofemoral pain: which are reliable and valid? Arch Phys Med Rehabil; 85:815–822.

[3] Paxton EW, Fithian DC, Stone ML, et al (2003) The reliability and validity of knee-specific and general health instruments in assessing acute patellar dislocation outcomes. Am J Sports Med; 31:487–492.

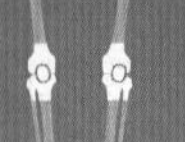

17. Kujala Patellofemoral Score (also know as the AKPS—Anterior Knee Pain Scale) (1993)

Details see previous pages.

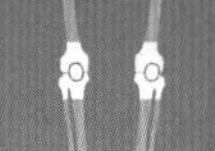

Methodological evaluation

 (5/6)

		no score	0 points	1 point	points
Validity	Content validity	not tested	not valid	**valid**	1
	Construct validity	not tested	not valid	**valid**	1
	Criterion validity	**not tested**	not valid	valid	-
Reliability	Internal consistency	not tested	not consistent	**consistent**	1
	Reproducibility	not tested	not reproducible	**reproducible**	1
	Responsiveness	not tested	not responsive	**responsive**	1
				Subtotal	**5**

Clinical utility

●●●○ (3/4)

	0 points	1 point	2 points	points
Patient friendliness	limited	**moderate**	strong	1
Clinician friendliness	limited	moderate	**strong**	2
			Subtotal	**3**

Total (out of 10) 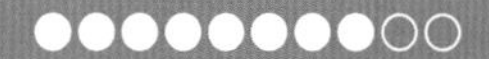 **8**

18. Lequesne - algofunctional index (1987)

Source: Lequesne MG, Mery C, Samson M, Gerard P (1987) Indexes of severity for osteoarthritis of the hip and knee. Validation--value in comparison with other assessment tests.
Scand J Rheumatol Suppl; 65:85–89.

Other versions available: German, Korean.

Content

Type Patient reported outcome
Scale 3 subscales (10 items):

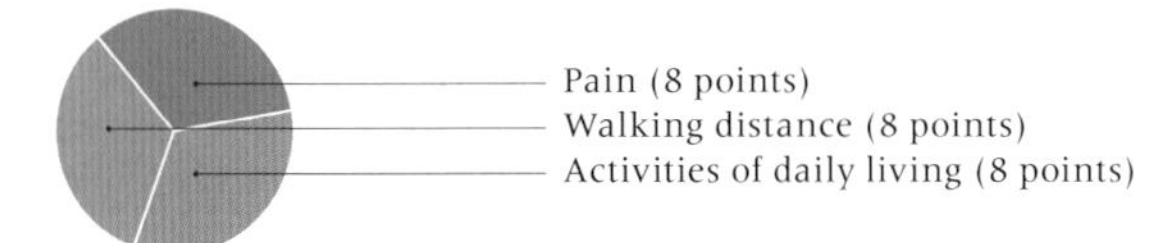

Interpretation
Handicap:
Extremely severe: > 13 points
Very severe: 11–13 points
Severe: 8–10 points
Moderate: 5–7 points
Minor: 1–4 points

Validation

Outcomes validated against [1]
- Pain
- Evaluator and patient opinion
- Timed stairs

Outcomes validated against [2]
- WOMAC
- X-rays
- Range of motion

Patient population tested in	Validity	Reliability	Responsiveness
Knee osteoarthritis (age NR; sex NR) [1]	+	+	not tested
Knee osteoarthritis (70 years; 33% male) [2]	+/-	+/-	not tested
Knee osteoarthritis (59 years; 8% male) [3]	+	+	+

Validation studies:

[1] Lequesne MG, Mery C, Samson M, et al (1987) Indexes of severity for osteoarthritis of the hip and knee. Validation--value in comparison with other assessment tests. Scand J Rheumatol Suppl; 65:85–89.
[2] Stucki G, Sangha O, Stucki S, et al (1998) Comparison of the WOMAC (Western Ontario and McMaster Universities) osteoarthritis index and a self-report format of the self-administered Lequesne-Algofunctional index in patients with knee and hip osteoarthritis. Osteoarthritis Cartilage; 6:79–86.
[3] Bae SC, Lee HS, Yun HR, et al (2001) Cross-cultural adaptation and validation of Korean Western Ontario and McMaster Universities (WOMAC) and Lequesne osteoarthritis indices for clinical research. Osteoarthritis Cartilage; 9:746–750.

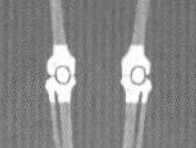

Methodological evaluation

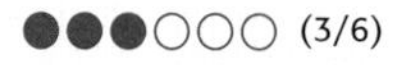 (3/6)

		no score	0 points	1 point	points
Validity	Content validity	not tested	not valid	valid	-
	Construct validity	not tested	not valid	valid	0
	Criterion validity	not tested	not valid	valid	1
Reliability	Internal consistency	not tested	not consistent	consistent	0
	Reproducibility	not tested	not reproducible	reproducible	1
	Responsiveness	not tested	not responsive	responsive	1
				Subtotal	**3**

Clinical utility

●●●● (4/4)

	0 points	1 point	2 points	points
Patient friendliness	limited	moderate	strong	2
Clinician friendliness	limited	moderate	strong	2
			Subtotal	**4**

Total (out of 10) 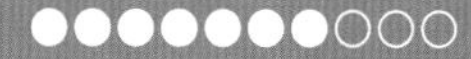 **7**

19. Lower Extremity Functional Scale (LEFS) (1999)

Source: Binkley JM, Stratford PW, Lott SA, Riddle DL (1999) The Lower Extremity Functional Scale (LEFS): scale development, measurement properties, and clinical application. North American Orthopaedic Rehabilitation Research Network.
Phys Ther; 79:371–383.

Content

Type Patient reported outcome
Scale

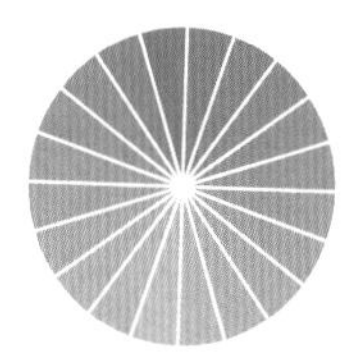

Functional activities:
20 questions (80 points)

Interpretation

Minimum score: 0 points
Maximum score: 80 points

The higher the score, the lower the function.

Validation

Outcomes validated against

- SF-36

Patient population tested in	Validity	Reliability	Responsiveness
Lower extremity dysfunction (44 years; 46% male)	+	+	+

Validation study:
Binkley JM, Stratford PW, Lott SA, et al (1999) The Lower Extremity Functional Scale (LEFS): scale development, measurement properties, and clinical application. North American Orthopaedic Rehabilitation Research Network. Phys Ther; 79:371–383.

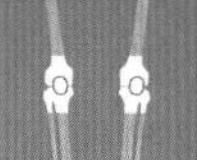

Methodological evaluation

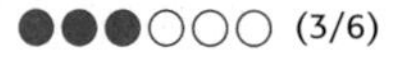 (3/6)

		no score	0 points	1 point	points
Validity	Content validity	not tested	not valid	valid	-
	Construct validity	not tested	not valid	valid	1
	Criterion validity	not tested	not valid	valid	-
Reliability	Internal consistency	not tested	not consistent	consistent	-
	Reproducibility	not tested	not reproducible	reproducible	1
	Responsiveness	not tested	not responsive	responsive	1
				Subtotal	**3**

Clinical utility

●●●○ (3/4)

	0 points	1 point	2 points	points
Patient friendliness	limited	moderate	strong	1
Clinician friendliness	limited	moderate	strong	2
			Subtotal	**3**

Total (out of 10) 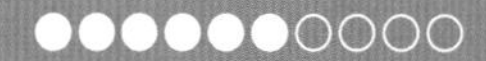 **6**

20. Lysholm knee function scoring scale (1982)

Sources: Lysholm J, Gillquist J (1982) Evaluation of knee ligament surgery results with special emphasis on use of a scoring scale. Am J Sports Med; 10:150–154.
Tegner Y, Lysholm J (1985) Rating systems in the evaluation of knee ligament injuries. Clin Orthop; (198):43–49.

Content

Type Patient reported outcome
Scale 8 subscales (8 items):

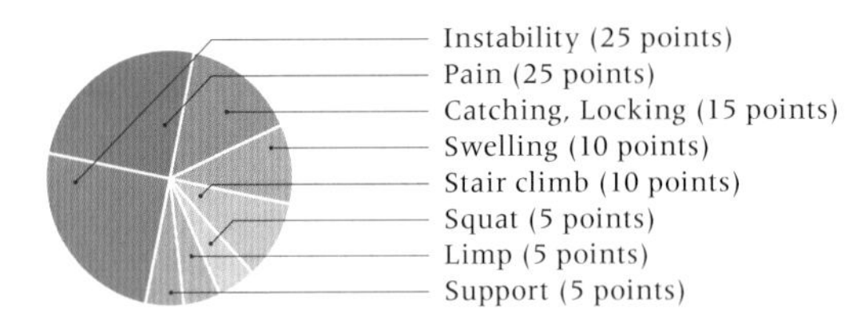

Interpretation

Excellent: 95–100 points
Good: 84–94 points
Fair: 65–83 points
Poor: < 65 points

Validation

Outcomes validated against [1]

- HSS knee scale
- Cincinnati knee rating system

Outcomes validated against [2]

- SF-36
- Cincinnati knee rating system
- Activites of daily living
- AAOS sports knee scale
- Patient rating
- Clinician rating

Outcomes validated against [3]

- Marshall scale

Outcomes validated against [4]

- Pain and global assessment

Validation (cont)

Patient population tested in	Validity	Reliability	Responsiveness
Anterior cruciate ligament surgery (25 years; sex NR) [1]	+	not tested	not tested
Athlete with variety of knee disorders (32 years; 52% male) [2]	+	+	+
Anterior cruciate ligament injury (27 years; 72% male) [3]	+	not tested	not tested
Variety of knee disorders (30 years; sex NR) [5]	not tested	+	not tested
Unstable knee (age NR; sex NR) [6]	not tested	+	not tested
Anterior cruciate ligament reconstruction (28 years; 53%male) [7]	not tested	not tested	-

Validation studies:

[1] Sgaglione NA, Del Pizzo W, Fox JM, et al (1995) Critical analysis of knee ligament rating systems. Am J Sports Med; 23:660–667.

[2] Marx RG, Jones EC, Allen AA, et al (2001) Reliability, validity, and responsiveness of four knee outcome scales for athletic patients. J Bone Joint Surg Am; 83-A:1459–1469.

[3] Tegner Y, Lysholm J (1985) Rating systems in the evaluation of knee ligament injuries. Clin Orthop; (198):43–49.

[4] Bae SC, Lee HS, Yun HR, et al (2001)Cross-cultural adaptation and validation of Korean Western Ontario and McMaster Universities (WOMAC) and Lequesne osteoarthritis indices for clinical research. Osteoarthritis Cartilage; 9:746–450.

[5] Bengtsson J, Mollborg J, Werner S (1996) A study for testing the sensitivity and reliability of the Lysholm knee scoring scale. Knee Surg Sports Traumatol Arthrosc; 4:27–31.

[6] Lysholm J, Gillquist J (1982) Evaluation of knee ligament surgery results with special emphasis on use of a scoring scale. Am J Sports Med; 10:150–154.

[7] Risberg MA, Holm I, Steen H, et al (1999) Sensitivity to changes over time for the IKDC form, the Lysholm score, and the Cincinnati knee score. A prospective study of 120 ACL reconstructed patients with a 2-year follow-up. Knee Surg Sports Traumatol Arthrosc; 7:152–159.

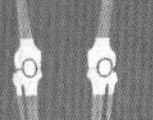

20. Lysholm knee function scoring scale (1982)

Details see previous pages.

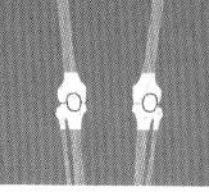

Methodological evaluation

●●●○○○ (3/6)

		no score	0 points	1 point	points
Validity	Content validity	not tested	not valid	valid	-
	Construct validity	not tested	not valid	valid	1
	Criterion validity	not tested	not valid	valid	1
Reliability	Internal consistency	not tested	not consistent	consistent	-
	Reproducibility	not tested	not reproducible	reproducible	1
	Responsiveness	not tested	not responsive	responsive	-
				Subtotal	**3**

Clinical utility

●●●● (4/4)

	0 points	1 point	2 points	points
Patient friendliness	limited	moderate	strong	2
Clinician friendliness	limited	moderate	strong	2
			Subtotal	**4**

Total (out of 10) ●●●●●●●○○○ **7**

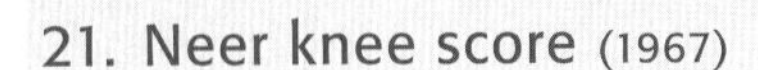

21. Neer knee score (1967)

Source: Neer CS 2nd, Grantham SA, Shelton ML (1967) Supracondylar fracture of the adult femur. A study of one hundred and ten cases. J Bone Joint Surg Am; 49:591–613.

Content

Type Clinician based outcome
Scale 6 subscales (6 items):

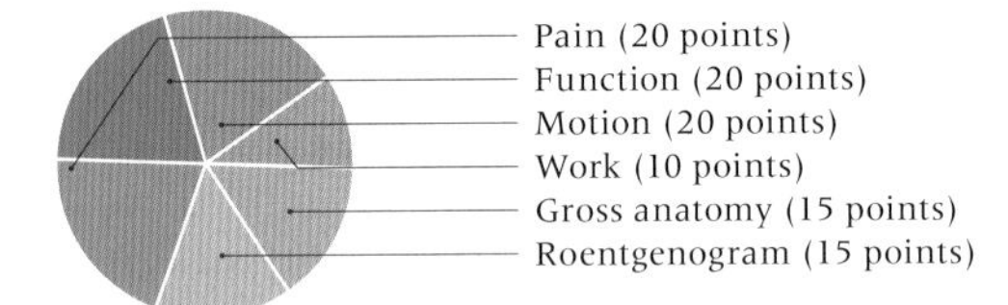

Interpretation

Excellent: 86–100 points
Satisfactory: 70–85 points
Unsatisfactory: 55–69 points
Failure: < 55 points

Validation

No validation studies were identified.

Patient population tested in	Validity	Reliability	Responsiveness
Not applicable			

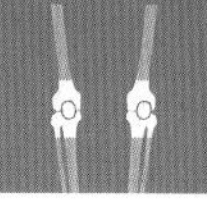

Methodological evaluation

○○○○○○ (0/6)

		no score	0 points	1 point	points
Validity	Content validity	not tested	not valid	valid	-
	Construct validity	not tested	not valid	valid	-
	Criterion validity	not tested	not valid	valid	-
Reliability	Internal consistency	not tested	not consistent	consistent	-
	Reproducibility	not tested	not reproducible	reproducible	-
	Responsiveness	not tested	not responsive	responsive	-
				Subtotal	-

Clinical utility

●●●○ (3/4)

	0 points	1 point	2 points	points
Patient friendliness	limited	moderate	strong	2
Clinician friendliness	limited	moderate	strong	1
			Subtotal	3

Total (out of 10) ●●●○○○○○○○ **3**

22. Oxford 12-item knee questionnaire (1998)

Source: Dawson J, Fitzpatrick R, Murray D, Carr A (1998) Questionnaire on the perceptions of patients about total knee replacement. J Bone Joint Surg Br; 80:63–69.

Other versions available: Swedish, Italian.

Content

Type Patient reported outcome

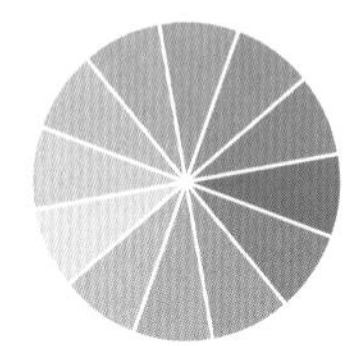

12 questions regarding perception of pain and function: 1–5 points for each.

Interpretation

Minimum score: 12 points; maximum score: 60 points
The higher the score, the lower the function.

Validation

Outcomes validated against [1]

- Health assesment questionnaire
- American knee society scoring system
- SF-36

Outcomes validated against [2]

- WOMAC
- NHP
- SF-12
- Sickness impact profile

Outcomes validated against [3]

- SF-36

Validation (cont)

Patient population tested in	Validity	Reliability	Responsiveness
Total knee arthroplasty (73 years; 44% male) [1]	+	+	+
Total knee arthroplasty (78 years; 30% male) [2]	+	+	+
Knee osteoarthritis (68 years; 38% male) [3]	+	+	not tested
Total knee arthroplasty (78 years; 30% male) [4]	not tested	+	+
Total knee arthroplasty (age NR; sex NR) [5]	not tested	+	+

Validation studies:

[1] Dawson J, Fitzpatrick R, Murray D, et al (1998) Questionnaire on the perceptions of patients about total knee replacement. J Bone Joint Surg Br; 80:63–69.

[2] Dunbar MJ, Robertsson O, Ryd L, et al (2000) Translation and validation of the Oxford-12 item knee score for use in Sweden. Acta Orthop Scand; 71:268–274, 2000.

[3] Padua R, Zanoli G, Ceccarelli E, et al (2003) The Italian version of the Oxford 12-item Knee Questionnaire-cross-cultural adaptation and validation. Int Orthop; 27(4):214–216.

[4] Dunbar MJ, Robertsson O, Ryd L, et al (2001) Appropriate questionnaires for knee arthroplasty. Results of a survey of 3600 patients from the Swedish Knee Arthroplasty Registry. J Bone Joint Surg Br; 83: 339–344.

[5] Liow RY, Walker K, Wajid MA, et al (2003) Functional rating for knee arthroplasty: comparison of three scoring systems. Orthopedics; 26: 143–149.

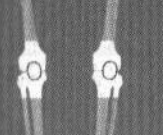

22. Oxford 12-item knee questionnaire (1998)

Details see previous pages.

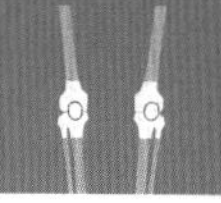

Methodological evaluation

●●●●●● (6/6)

		no score	0 points	1 point	points
Validity	Content validity	not tested	not valid	valid	1
	Construct validity	not tested	not valid	valid	1
	Criterion validity	not tested	not valid	valid	1
Reliability	Internal consistency	not tested	not consistent	consistent	1
	Reproducibility	not tested	not reproducible	reproducible	1
	Responsiveness	not tested	not responsive	responsive	1
				Subtotal	**6**

Clinical utility

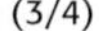 (3/4)

	0 points	1 point	2 points	points
Patient friendliness	limited	moderate	strong	1
Clinician friendliness	limited	moderate	strong	2
			Subtotal	**3**

Total (out of 10)  **9**

23. Rheumatoid and Arthritis Outcome Score for the lower extremity (RAOS) (2003)

Source: Bremander AB, Petersson IF, Roos EM (2004) Validation of the Rheumatoid and Arthritis Outcome Score (RAOS) for the lower extremity.
Health Qual Life Outcomes; 1:55.

Adaptation to the KOOS.

Content

Type Patient reported outcome
Scale 5 subscales (42 items):

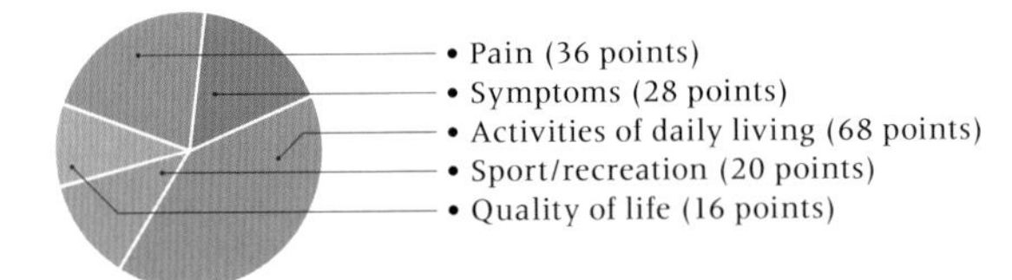

Likert scale for each item (5 choices).

Interpretation

Scores normalized to 100 for each subscale and each subscale scored separately.

The higher the score, the higher the function.

Validation

Outcomes validated against

- Health assessment questionnaire
- SF-36
- Arthritis impact measurement scale

Patient population tested in	Validity	Reliability	Responsiveness
Patients with chronic inflammatory joint disease (56 years; 27% male)	+	+	+

Validation study:
Bremander AB, Petersson IF, Roos EM (2004) Validation of the Rheumatoid and Arthritis Outcome Score (RAOS) for the lower extremity. Health Qual Life Outcomes; 1:55.

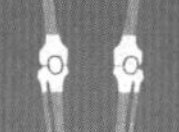

Methodological evaluation

 (5/6)

		no score	0 points	1 point	points
Validity	Content validity	not tested	not valid	valid	1
	Construct validity	not tested	not valid	valid	1
	Criterion validity	not tested	not valid	valid	-
Reliability	Internal consistency	not tested	not consistent	consistent	1
	Reproducibility	not tested	not reproducible	reproducible	1
	Responsiveness	not tested	not responsive	responsive	1
				Subtotal	**5**

Clinical utility

●●○○ (2/4)

	0 points	1 point	2 points	points
Patient friendliness	limited	moderate	strong	0
Clinician friendliness	limited	moderate	strong	2
			Subtotal	**2**

Total (out of 10) 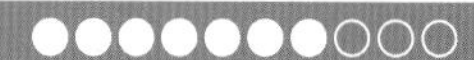 **7**

24. Single Assessment Numeric Evaluation (SANE) (2000)

Source: Williams GN, Taylor DC, Gangel TJ, Uhorchak JM, Arciero RA (2000) Comparison of the single assessment numeric evaluation method and the Lysholm score.
Clin Orthop; 373:184–192.

Content

Type Patient reported outcome
Scale

Single question:
"On a scale of 0 to 100, how would you rate your knee function with 100 being normal?"

Interpretation

Minimum score: 0 points
Maximum score: 100 points

The higher the score, the higher the function.

Validation

Outcomes validated against

- Modified Lysholm knee function scoring scale

Patient population tested in	Validity	Reliability	Responsiveness
Anterior cruciate ligament reconstruction (21 years; 83% male)	+	not tested	+

Validation study:

Williams GN, Taylor DC, Gangel TJ, et al (2000) Comparison of the single assessment numeric evaluation method and the Lysholm score. Clin Orthop; 373:184–192.

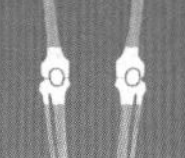

Methodological evaluation

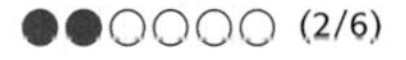 (2/6)

		no score	0 points	1 point	points
Validity	Content validity	**not tested**	not valid	valid	-
	Construct validity	**not tested**	not valid	valid	-
	Criterion validity	not tested	not valid	**valid**	1
Reliability	Internal consistency	**not tested**	not consistent	consistent	-
	Reproducibility	**not tested**	not reproducible	reproducible	-
	Responsiveness	not tested	not responsive	**responsive**	1
				Subtotal	**2**

Clinical utility

●●●● (4/4)

	0 points	1 point	2 points	points
Patient friendliness	limited	moderate	**strong**	2
Clinician friendliness	limited	moderate	**strong**	2
			Subtotal	**4**

Total (out of 10) 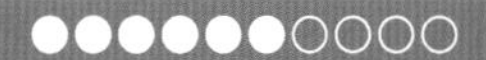 **6**

25. Tegner activity level rating scale (1985)

Source: Tegner Y, Lysholm J (1985) Rating systems in the evaluation of knee ligament injuries.
Clin Orthop; (198):43–49.

Content

Type Patient reported outcome
Scale

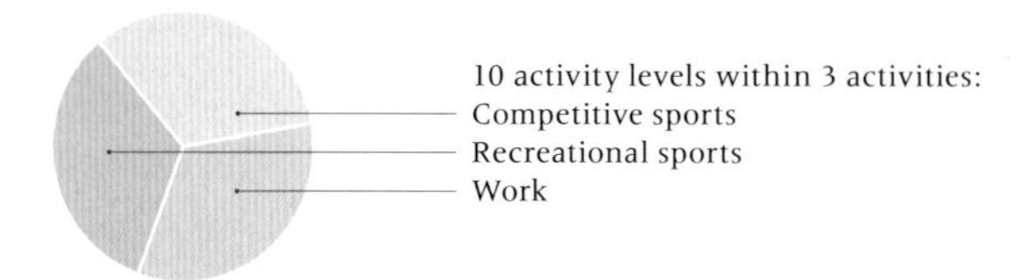

Interpretation

Minimum score : 0 points (sick leave or disability pension)
Maximum: 10 points (national and international elite soccer)

Validation

Outcomes validated against

- Early Lysholm knee function scoring scale

Patient population tested in	Validity	Reliability	Responsiveness
Anterior cruciate ligament injury (27 years; 72% male)	+	not tested	not tested

Validation study:

Wegner Y, Lysholm J (1985) Rating systems in the evaluation of knee ligament injuries. Clin Orthop; (198):43–49.

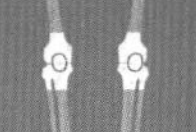

Methodological evaluation

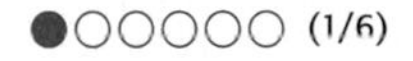 (1/6)

		no score	0 points	1 point	points
Validity	Content validity	not tested	not valid	valid	-
	Construct validity	not tested	not valid	valid	-
	Criterion validity	not tested	not valid	valid	1
Reliability	Internal consistency	not tested	not consistent	consistent	-
	Reproducibility	not tested	not reproducible	reproducible	-
	Responsiveness	not tested	not responsive	responsive	-
				Subtotal	1

Clinical utility

●●●● (4/4)

	0 points	1 point	2 points	points
Patient friendliness	limited	moderate	strong	2
Clinician friendliness	limited	moderate	strong	2
			Subtotal	4

Total (out of 10) 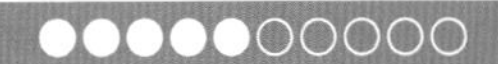 **5**

26. Western Ontario and McMaster Universities OA index (WOMAC) (1988)

Source: Bellamy N, Buchanan WW, Goldsmith CH, Campbell J, Stitt LW (1988) Validation study of WOMAC: a health status instrument for measuring clinically important patient relevant outcomes to antirheumatic drug therapy in patients with osteoarthritis of the hip or knee. J Rheumatol; 15:1833–1840.

Other versions available: computerized, German, Hebrew, Swedish, Korean.

Content

Type Patient reported outcome
Scale 3 subscales (24 items):

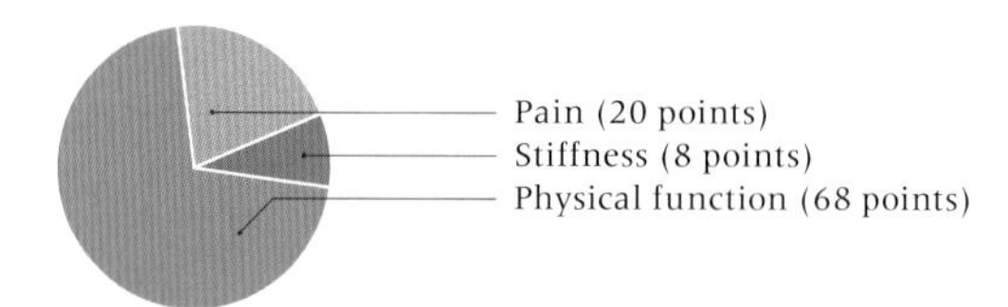

Interpretation

Minimum score: 0 points
Maximum score: 96 points

The higher the score, the lower the function.

Validation

Outcomes validated against [1]

- Lequesne - algofunctional index
- Doyle index
- McMaster health index

Outcomes validated against [2]

- Paper version of the WOMAC

Outcomes validated against [3]

- VAS for pain and handicap

Outcomes validated against [4]

- SF-36
- Radiographic OA

Outcomes validated against [5]

- Pain and global assessment

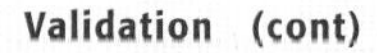

Validation (cont)

Patient population tested in	Validity	Reliability	Responsiveness
Total knee arthroplasty (67 years; 46% male) [1]	+	+	+
Knee osteoarthritis (65 years; 37% male) [2]	+	not tested	not tested
Knee osteoarthritis (age NR; 15% male) [3]	+	+	not tested
Knee cartilage damage (48 years; 27% male) [4]	+	not tested	+
Knee cartilage damage (age NR; sex NR) [4]	not tested	+	not tested
Knee osteoarthritis (59 years; 8% male) [5]	+	+	+
Knee osteoarthritis (55 years; 20% male) [6]	+	+	not tested
Total knee arthroplasty (78 years; 30% male) [7]	not tested	+	not tested
Knee osteoarthritis (70 years; 33% male) [8]	+	+	not tested

Validation studies:

[1] Bellamy N, Buchanan WW, Goldsmith CH, et al (1988) Validation study of WOMAC: a health status instrument for measuring clinically important patient relevant outcomes to antirheumatic drug therapy in patients with osteoarthritis of the hip or knee. J Rheumatol; 15: 1833–1840.

[2] Bellamy N, Campbell J, Stevens J, et al (1997) Validation study of a computerized version of the Western Ontario and McMaster Universities VA3.0 Osteoarthritis Index. J Rheumatol; 24:2413–2415.

[3] Wigler I, Neumann L, Yaron M (1999) Validation study of a Hebrew version of WOMAC in patients with osteoarthritis of the knee. Clin Rheumatol; 18:402–405.

[4] Roos EM, Klassbo M, Lohmander LS (1999) WOMAC osteoarthritis index. Reliability, validity, and responsiveness in patients with arthroscopically assessed osteoarthritis. Western Ontario and MacMaster Universities. Scand J Rheumatol; 28:210–215.

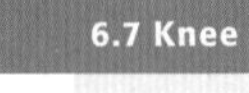

26. Western Ontario and McMaster Universities OA index (WOMAC) (1988)

Details see previous pages.

Validation (cont)

[5] Bae SC, Lee HS, Yun HR, et al (2001) Cross-cultural adaptation and validation of Korean Western Ontario and McMaster Universities (WOMAC) and Lequesne osteoarthritis indices for clinical research. Osteoarthritis Cartilage; 9:746–750.
[6] Thumboo J, Chew LH, Soh CH (2001) Validation of the Western Ontario and Mcmaster University osteoarthritis index in Asians with osteoarthritis in Singapore.
Osteoarthritis Cartilage; 9:440–446.
[7] Dunbar MJ, Robertsson O, Ryd L, et al (2001) Appropriate questionnaires for knee arthroplasty. Results of a survey of 3600 patients from The Swedish Knee Arthroplasty Registry. J Bone Joint Surg Br; 83:339–344.
[8] Stucki G, Sangha O, Stucki S, et al (1998) Comparison of the WOMAC (Western Ontario and McMaster Universities) osteoarthritis index and a self-report format of the self-administered Lequesne-Algofunctional index in patients with knee and hip osteoarthritis. Osteoarthritis Cartilage; 6:79–86.

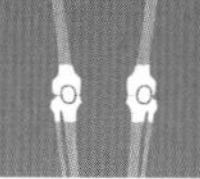

Methodological evaluation ●●●●●● (6/6)

		no score	0 points	1 point	points
Validity	Content validity	not tested	not valid	valid	1
	Construct validity	not tested	not valid	valid	1
	Criterion validity	not tested	not valid	valid	1
Reliability	Internal consistency	not tested	not consistent	consistent	1
	Reproducibility	not tested	not reproducible	reproducible	1
	Responsiveness	not tested	not responsive	responsive	1
				Subtotal	6

Clinical utility ●●○○ (2/4)

	0 points	1 point	2 points	points
Patient friendliness	limited	moderate	strong	0
Clinician friendliness	limited	moderate	strong	2
			Subtotal	2

Total (out of 10)  **8**

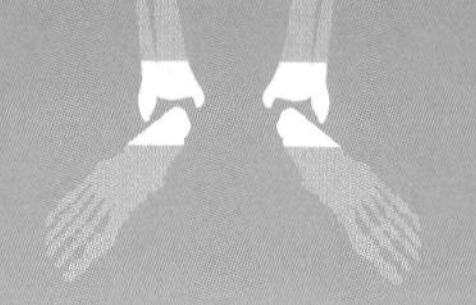

6.8 Ankle

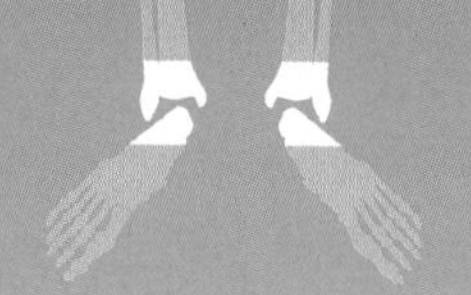

1. AAOS foot and ankle core score

Source: AAOS Normative Data Study and Outcomes Instruments: American Academy of Orthopaedic Surgeons
http://www.aaos.org

Content

Type Patient reported outcome
Scale 4 subscales (20 items):

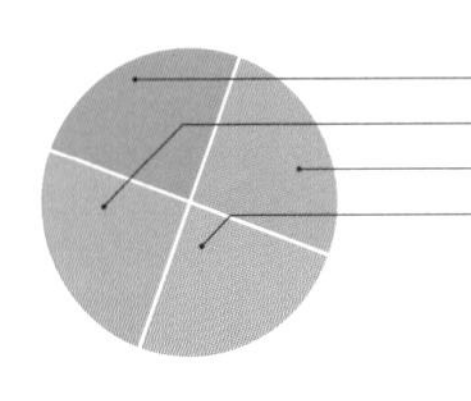

20 questions relating to:
Pain (9 items)
Function (6 items)
Stiffness and swelling(2 items)
Giving way (3 items)

A shoe comfort scale (5 questions) can be administered as a companion to the foot and ankle core score.

Interpretation

Each subscale is scored separately and normalized to 100.

The higher the score, the higher the function

Validation

Outcomes validated against

- AAOS lower limb core scale
- SF-36
- Physician assessment

Patient population tested in	Validity	Reliability	Responsiveness
Patients with foot or ankle complaints (54% male; 48 years)	+	+	+

Validation study:
Johanson NA, Liang MH, Daltroy L, et al (2004) American Academy of Orthopaedic Surgeons lower limb outcomes assessment instruments. Reliability, validity, and sensitivity to change. J Bone Joint Surg Am; 86-A:902–909.

Methodological evaluation

 (5/6)

		no score	0 points	1 point	points
Validity	Content validity	not tested	not valid	valid	1
	Construct validity	not tested	not valid	valid	1
	Criterion validity	not tested	not valid	valid	-
Reliability	Internal consistency	not tested	not consistent	consistent	1
	Reproducibility	not tested	not reproducible	reproducible	1
	Responsiveness	not tested	not responsive	responsive	1
				Subtotal	**5**

Clinical utility

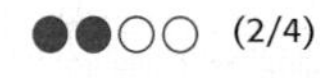 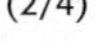 (2/4)

	0 points	1 point	2 points	points
Patient friendliness	limited	moderate	strong	0
Clinician friendliness	limited	moderate	strong	2
			Subtotal	**2**

Total (out of 10) 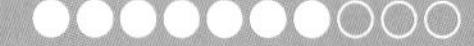 **7**

2. Ankle-hindfoot scale of the American Orthopaedic Foot and Ankle Society (1994)

Source: Kitaoka HB, Alexander IJ, Adelaar RS, Nunley JA, Myerson MS, Sanders M (1994) Clinical rating systems for the ankle-hindfoot, midfoot, hallux, and lesser toes.
Foot Ankle Int; 15:349–353.

Content

Type Clinician based outcome
Scale 3 subscales (9 items):

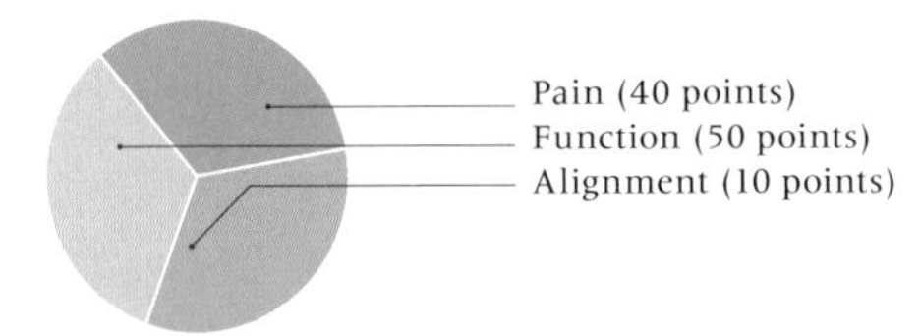

Interpretation

Minimum score: 0 points
Maximum score: 100 points

The higher the score, the higher the function.

Validation

Outcomes validated against

- SF-36

Patient population tested in	Validity	Reliability	Responsiveness
Patients presenting with ankle complaints (50 years; 42% male)	+/-	-	not tested

Validation study:
SooHoo NF, Shuler M, Fleming LL (2003) Evaluation of the validity of the AOFAS Clinical Rating Systems by correlation to the SF-36. Foot Ankle Int; 24:50–55.

Methodological evaluation ●○○○○○ (1/6)

		no score	0 points	1 point	points
Validity	Content validity	not tested	not valid	**valid**	1
Validity	Construct validity	not tested	**not valid**	valid	0
Validity	Criterion validity	**not tested**	not valid	valid	-
Reliability	Internal consistency	**not tested**	not consistent	consistent	-
Reliability	Reproducibility	not tested	**not reproducible**	reproducible	0
	Responsiveness	**not tested**	not responsive	responsive	-
				Subtotal	1

Clinical utility ●●●● (4/4)

	0 points	1 point	2 points	points
Patient friendliness	limited	moderate	**strong**	2
Clinician friendliness	limited	moderate	**strong**	2
			Subtotal	4

Total (out of 10) 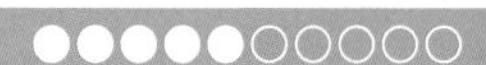 **5**

3. Ankle Joint Functional Assessment Tool (AJFAT) (1999)

Source: Rozzi SL, Lephart SM, Sterner R, Kuligowski L (1999) Balance training for persons with functionally unstable ankles.
J Orthop Sports Phys Ther; 29:478–486.

Content

Type Patient related outcome
Scale 5 subscales (12 items):

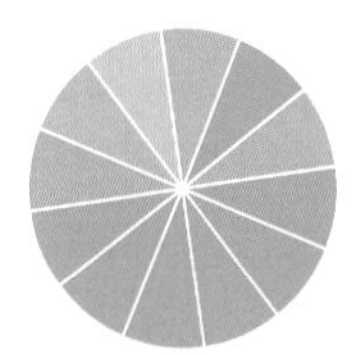

12 questions (0 to 4 points each) relating to: Pain, strength, stability, swelling, and activities.

Interpretation

Minimum score: 0 points
Maximum score: 48 points

The higher the score, the higher the function.

Validation

No validation studies were identified.

Patient population tested in	Validity	Reliability	Responsiveness
Not applicable			

3. Ankle Joint Functional Assessment Tool (AJFAT) (1999)

Methodological evaluation

○○○○○○ (0/6)

		no score	0 points	1 point	points
Validity	Content validity	not tested	not valid	valid	-
	Construct validity	not tested	not valid	valid	-
	Criterion validity	not tested	not valid	valid	-
Reliability	Internal consistency	not tested	not consistent	consistent	-
	Reproducibility	not tested	not reproducible	reproducible	-
	Responsiveness	not tested	not responsive	responsive	-
				Subtotal	-

Clinical utility

●●●○ (3/4)

	0 points	1 point	2 points	points
Patient friendliness	limited	moderate	strong	1
Clinician friendliness	limited	moderate	strong	2
			Subtotal	3

Total (out of 10) 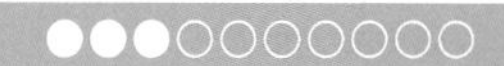 **3**

4. Ankle osteoarthritis score (2003) (modification of the foot function index)

Source: Domsic RT, Saltzman CL (1998) Ankle osteoarthritis scale. Foot Ankle Int; 19:466–471.

Content

Type Patient reported outcome
Scale 2 subscales (18 items):

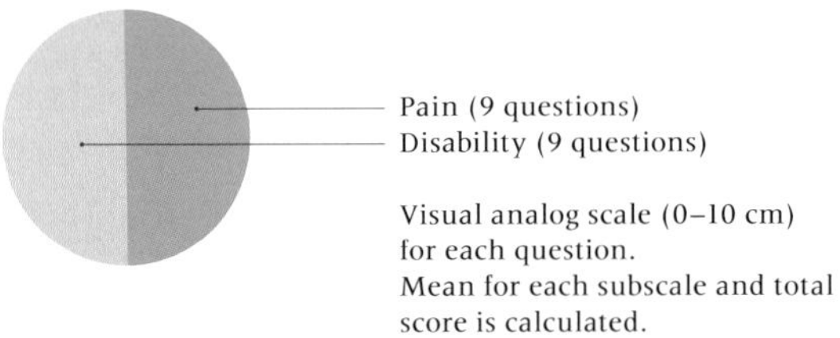

Interpretation

Scores are normalized to 100 for each subscale and total score.
Minimum score: 0 points
Maximum score: 100 points

The higher the score, the lower the function.

Validation

Outcomes validated against

- SF-36
- WOMAC
- Single leg heel lifts

Patient population tested in	Validity	Reliability	Responsiveness
Isolated osteoarthritis of the ankle (52.7 years; 57% male)	+	+	not tested

Validation study:
Domsic RT, Saltzman CL (1998) Ankle osteoarthritis scale. Foot Ankle Int; 19:466–471.

4. Ankle osteoarthritis score (2003) (modification of the foot function index)

Methodological evaluation

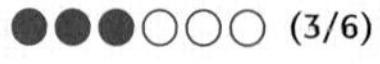
(3/6)

		no score	0 points	1 point	points
Validity	Content validity	not tested	not valid	valid	-
	Construct validity	not tested	not valid	valid	1
	Criterion validity	not tested	not valid	valid	1
Reliability	Internal consistency	not tested	not consistent	consistent	-
	Reproducibility	not tested	not reproducible	reproducible	1
	Responsiveness	not tested	not responsive	responsive	-
				Subtotal	**3**

Clinical utility

●●●○ (3/4)

	0 points	1 point	2 points	points
Patient friendliness	limited	moderate	strong	1
Clinician friendliness	limited	moderate	strong	2
			Subtotal	**3**

Total (out of 10)  **6**

5. Ankle-rating scale of Kaikkonen (1994)

Source: Kaikkonen A, Kannus P, Jarvinen M (1994) A performance test protocol and scoring scale for the evaluation of ankle injuries. Am J Sports Med; 22:462–469.

Content

Type Clinician based outcome
Scale 6 subscales (9 items):

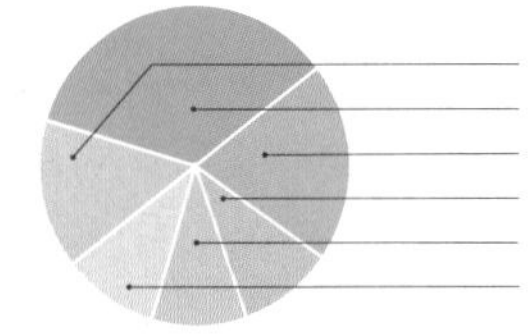

Interpretation
Excellent: 85–100 points
Good: 70–84 points
Fair: 55–69 points
Poor: < 54 points

Validation

Outcomes validated against
- Walking down staircase
- Heel and toe raises
- Balance test
- Range of motion
- Isokinetic evaluation
- Subjective opinion

Patient population tested in	Validity	Reliability	Responsiveness
Operatively treated grade III lateral ligament injury of the ankle (36 years; 61% male)	+	+*	+

Validation study:
Kaikkonen A, Kannus P, Jarvinen M (1994) A performance test protocol and scoring scale for the evaluation of ankle injuries. Am J Sports Med; 22:462–469.

** Reliability testing was performed in a noninjured reference population.*

Methodological evaluation

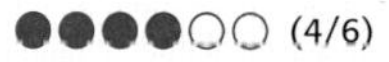
(4/6)

		no score	0 points	1 point	points
Validity	Content validity	not tested	not valid	**valid**	1
	Construct validity	not tested	not valid	**valid**	1
	Criterion validity	**not tested**	not valid	valid	-
Reliability	Internal consistency	**not tested**	not consistent	consistent	-
	Reproducibility	not tested	not reproducible	**reproducible**	1
	Responsiveness	not tested	not responsive	**responsive**	1
				Subtotal	**4**

Clinical utility

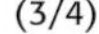
(3/4)

	0 points	1 point	2 points	points
Patient friendliness	limited	moderate	**strong**	2
Clinician friendliness	limited	**moderate**	strong	1
			Subtotal	**3**

Total (out of 10) 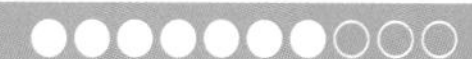 **7**

6. Foot and ankle outcome score (2001)

Source: Roos EM, Brandsson S, Karlsson J (2001) Validation of the foot and ankle outcome score for ankle ligament reconstruction. Foot Ankle Int; 22:788–794.

Content

Type Patient reported outcome
Scale 5 subscales (42 items):

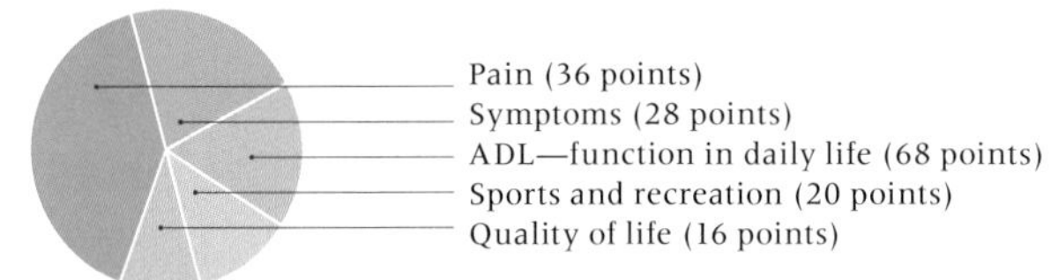

5-point Likert scale for each question.

Interpretation

Scores normalized to 100 for each subscale and each subscale scored separately.

Minimum subscale score: 0 points
Maximum subscale score: 100 points

The higher the score, the higher the function.

Validation

Outcomes validated against

- Karlsson ankle score

Patient population tested in	Validity	Reliability	Responsiveness
Patients with anatomical reconstruction of lateral ankle ligaments (39.6 years; 60% male)	+	+	not tested

Validation study:
Roos EM, Brandsson S, Karlsson J (2001) Validation of the foot and ankle outcome score for ankle ligament reconstruction. Foot Ankle Int; 22:788–794.

6. Foot and ankle outcome score (2001)

Methodological evaluation

●●●●○○ (4/6)

		no score	0 points	1 point	points
Validity	Content validity	not tested	not valid	**valid**	1
Validity	Construct validity	not tested	not valid	**valid**	1
Validity	Criterion validity	**not tested**	not valid	valid	-
Reliability	Internal consistency	not tested	not consistent	**consistent**	1
Reliability	Reproducibility	not tested	not reproducible	**reproducible**	1
	Responsiveness	**not tested**	not responsive	responsive	-
				Subtotal	**4**

Clinical utility

●●○○ (2/4)

	0 points	1 point	2 points	points
Patient friendliness	**limited**	moderate	strong	0
Clinician friendliness	limited	moderate	**strong**	2
			Subtotal	**2**

Total (out of 10) 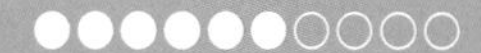 **6**

7. Foot function index (1991)

Source: Budiman-Mak E, Conrad KJ, Roach KE (1991) The Foot Function Index: a measure of foot pain and disability. J Clin Epidemiol; 44:561–570.

Content

Type Patient reported outcome
Scale 3 subscales (23 items):

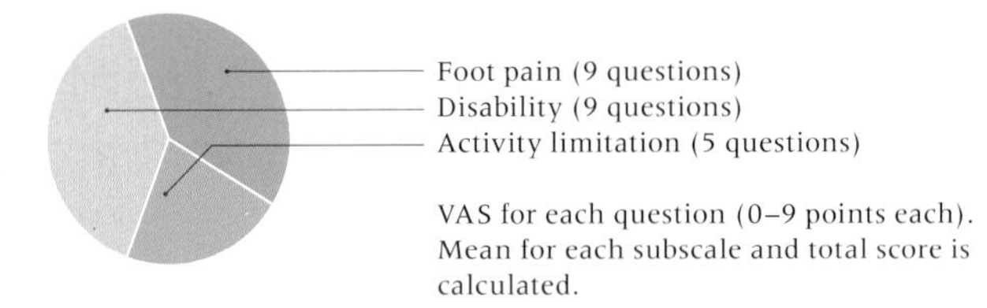

VAS for each question (0–9 points each). Mean for each subscale and total score is calculated.

Interpretation
Scores normalized to 100 for each subscale and total score.

Minimum score: 0 points
Maximum score: 100 points

The higher the score, the lower the function.

Validation

Outcomes validated against
- Foot joint count
- 50 feet walking time
- Foot grip strength

Patient population tested in	Validity	Reliability	Responsiveness
Definite or classical rheumatoid arthritis (61 years; 89% male)	+	+	+

Validation study:
Budiman-Mak E, Conrad KJ, Roach KE (1991) The Foot Function Index: a measure of foot pain and disability. J Clin Epidemiol; 44:561–570.

Methodological evaluation

●●●●●○ (5/6)

		no score	0 points	1 point	points
Validity	Content validity	not tested	not valid	valid	-
	Construct validity	not tested	not valid	valid	1
	Criterion validity	not tested	not valid	valid	1
Reliability	Internal consistency	not tested	not consistent	consistent	1
	Reproducibility	not tested	not reproducible	reproducible	1
	Responsiveness	not tested	not responsive	responsive	1
				Subtotal	**5**

Clinical utility

●●○○ (2/4)

	0 points	1 point	2 points	points
Patient friendliness	limited	moderate	strong	0
Clinician friendliness	limited	moderate	strong	2
			Subtotal	**2**

Total (out of 10) 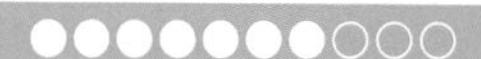 **7**

8. Foot health status questionnaire (1998)

Source: Bennett PJ, Patterson C, Wearing S, Baglioni T (1998)
Development and validation of a questionnaire designed to measure foot-health status.
J Am Podiatr Med Assoc; 88:419–428.

Content

Type Patient reported outcome
Scale 4 subscales (13 items):

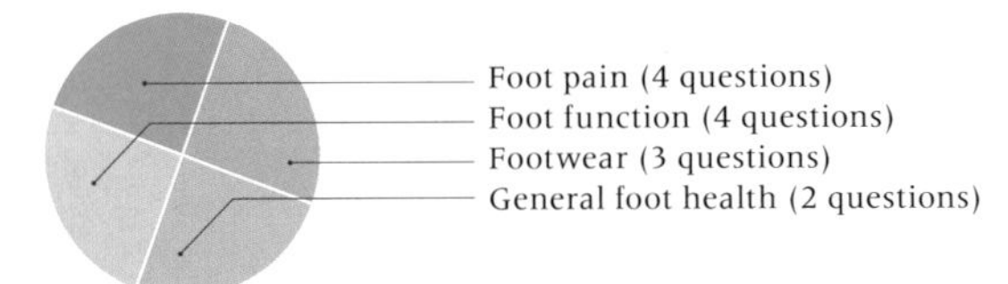

Interpretation

Each subscale normalized to 100; each subscale scored separately.

Minimum score: 0 points
Maximum score: 100 points

The higher the score, the higher the function.

Validation

Outcomes validated against

- Foot function Index
- Classification of foot diagnoses (minor pathology, acute disease, morphological problems)

Patient population tested in	Validity	Reliability	Responsiveness
Adult volunteers with various foot complaints who were visiting a podiatric clinic	+	+	+

Validation study:
Bennett PJ, Patterson C, Wearing S, Baglioni T (1998) Development and validation of a questionnaire designed to measure foot-health status.
J Am Podiatr Med Assoc; 88:419–428.

Methodological evaluation

(G/G)

		no score	0 points	1 point	points
Validity	Content validity	not tested	not valid	valid	1
	Construct validity	not tested	not valid	valid	1
	Criterion validity	not tested	not valid	valid	1
Reliability	Internal consistency	not tested	not consistent	consistent	1
	Reproducibility	not tested	not reproducible	reproducible	1
	Responsiveness	not tested	not responsive	responsive	1
				Subtotal	**6**

Clinical utility

(3/4)

	0 points	1 point	2 points	points
Patient friendliness	limited	moderate	strong	1
Clinician friendliness	limited	moderate	strong	2
			Subtotal	**3**

Total (out of 10) 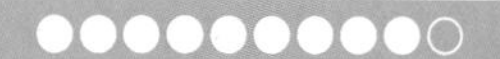 **9**

9. Freiburg ankle score (1998)

Source: Lahm A, Erggelet C, Steinwachs M, Reichelt A (1998) Arthroscopic therapy of osteochondrosis dissecans of the talus–follow-up with a new "Ankle Score". Sportverletz Sportschaden; 12:107–113.

Content

Type Clinician based outcome
Scale 7 subscales (8 items):

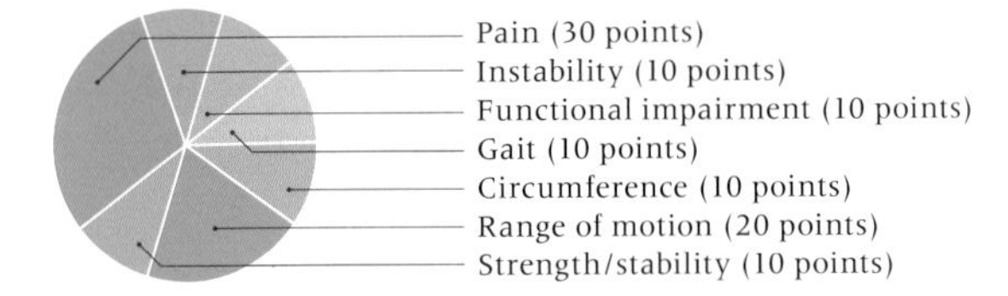

Interpretation

Minimum score: 0 points
Maximum score: 100 points

The higher the score, the higher the function.

Validation

No validation studies were identified.

Patient population tested in	Validity	Reliability	Responsiveness
Not applicable			

Methodological evaluation ○○○○○○ (0/6)

		no score	0 points	1 point	points
Validity	Content validity	not tested	not valid	valid	-
	Construct validity	not tested	not valid	valid	-
	Criterion validity	not tested	not valid	valid	-
Reliability	Internal consistency	not tested	not consistent	consistent	-
	Reproducibility	not tested	not reproducible	reproducible	-
	Responsiveness	not tested	not responsive	responsive	-
				Subtotal	-

Clinical utility ●●○○ (2/4)

	0 points	1 point	2 points	points
Patient friendliness	limited	moderate	strong	0
Clinician friendliness	limited	moderate	strong	2
			Subtotal	2

Total (out of 10) 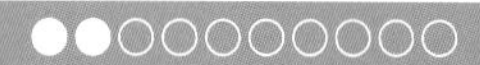 **2**

10. Good, Jones, and Lingstone grading system of lateral ankle stability (1975)

Source: Good CJ, Jones MA, Lingstone BN (1975) Reconstruction of the lateral ligament of the ankle.
Injury; 7:63–65.

Content

Type Clinician based outcome
Scale 5 subscales:

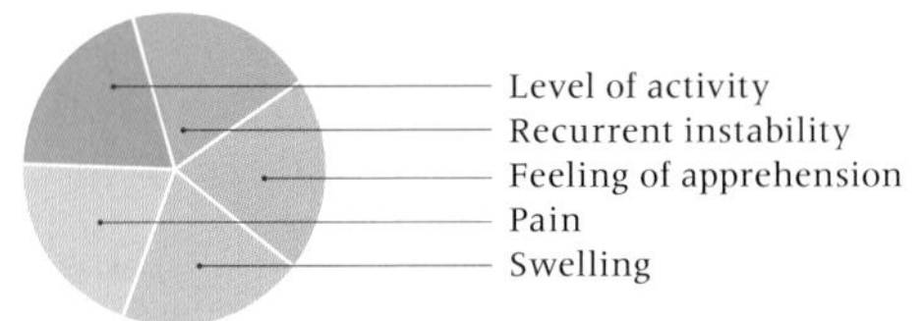

A combination of these criteria fit into 1 of 4 grades (grade 1, grade 2, grade 3, and grade 4).

Interpretation

The higher the grade, the higher the function.

Validation

No validation studies were identified.

Patient population tested in	Validity	Reliability	Responsiveness
Not applicable			

10. Good, Jones, and Lingstone grading system of lateral ankle stability (1975)

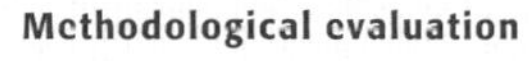

Methodological evaluation

○○○○○○ (0/6)

		no score	0 points	1 point	points
Validity	Content validity	not tested	not valid	valid	-
	Construct validity	not tested	not valid	valid	-
	Criterion validity	not tested	not valid	valid	-
Reliability	Internal consistency	not tested	not consistent	consistent	-
	Reproducibility	not tested	not reproducible	reproducible	-
	Responsiveness	not tested	not responsive	responsive	-
				Subtotal	-

Clinical utility

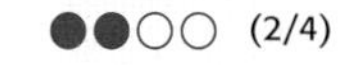

●●○○ (2/4)

	0 points	1 point	2 points	points
Patient friendliness	limited	moderate	strong	0
Clinician friendliness	limited	moderate	strong	2
			Subtotal	2

Total (out of 10)

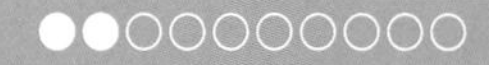

●●○○○○○○○○ **2**

11. Hallux metatarsophalangeal-interphalangeal score of the American Orthopaedic Foot and Ankle Society (1994)

Source: Kitaoka HB, Alexander IJ, Adelaar RS, Nunley JA, Myerson MS, Sanders M (1994) Clinical rating systems for the ankle-hindfoot, midfoot, hallux, and lesser toes.
Foot Ankle Int; 15:349–353.

Content

Type Clinician based outcome
Scale 3 subscales (8 items):

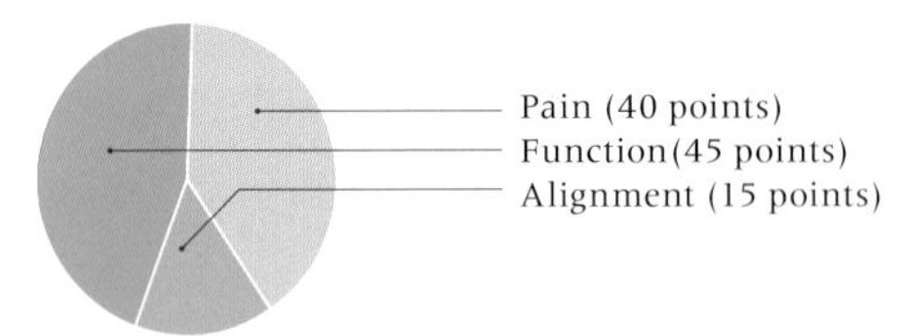

Interpretation

Minimum score: 0 points
Maximum score: 100 points

The higher the score, the higher the function.

Validation

Outcomes validated against

- SF-36

Patient population tested in	Validity	Reliability	Responsiveness
Patients presenting with ankle complaints (50 years; 42% male)	+/-	-	not tested

Validation study:

SooHoo NF, Shuler M, Fleming LL (2003) Evaluation of the validity of the AOFAS Clinical Rating Systems by correlation to the SF-36.
Foot Ankle Int; 24:50–55.

Methodological evaluation

●○○○○○ (1/6)

		no score	0 points	1 point	points
Validity	Content validity	not tested	not valid	**valid**	1
	Construct validity	not tested	**not valid**	valid	0
	Criterion validity	**not tested**	not valid	valid	-
Reliability	Internal consistency	**not tested**	not consistent	consistent	-
	Reproducibility	not tested	**not reproducible**	reproducible	0
	Responsiveness	**not tested**	not responsive	responsive	-
				Subtotal	**1**

Clinical utility

(4/4)

	0 points	1 point	2 points	points
Patient friendliness	limited	moderate	**strong**	2
Clinician friendliness	limited	moderate	**strong**	2
			Subtotal	**4**

Total (out of 10)

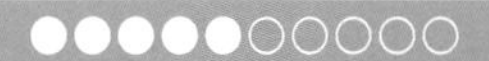

5

12. Iowa ankle score (1989)

Source: Merchant TC, Dietz FR (1989) Long-term follow-up after fractures of the tibial and fibular shafts.
J Bone Joint Surg Am; 71:599–606.

Content

Type Clinician based outcome
Scale 4 subscales (10 items):

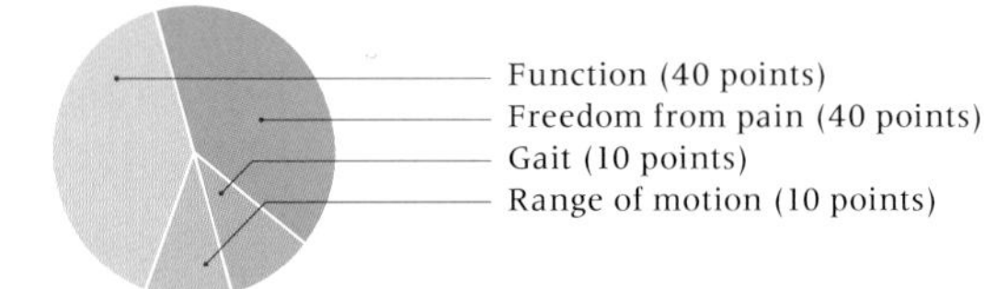

Interpretation
Excellent: 90–100 points
Good: 80–89 points
Fair: 70–79 points
Poor: < 70 points

Validation

Outcomes validated against
- SF-36

Patient population tested in	Validity	Reliability	Responsiveness
Tibial shaft fractures treated with closed intramedullary nailing (43 years; 72% male)	+	not tested	not tested

Validation study:
Dogra AS, Ruiz AL, Marsh DR (2002) Late outcome of isolated tibial fractures treated by intramedullary nailing: the correlation between disease-specific and generic outcome measures. J Orthop Trauma; 16:245–249.

Methodological evaluation

●○○○○○ (1/6)

		no score	0 points	1 point	points
Validity	Content validity	not tested	not valid	valid	-
	Construct validity	not tested	not valid	valid	1
	Criterion validity	not tested	not valid	valid	-
Reliability	Internal consistency	not tested	not consistent	consistent	-
	Reproducibility	not tested	not reproducible	reproducible	-
	Responsiveness	not tested	not responsive	responsive	-
				Subtotal	1

Clinical utility

●●●○ (3/4)

	0 points	1 point	2 points	points
Patient friendliness	limited	moderate	strong	2
Clinician friendliness	limited	moderate	strong	1
			Subtotal	3

Total (out of 10) ●●●●○○○○○○ **4**

13. Karlsson Ankle Function Score (KAFS) (1991)

Source: Karlsson J (1991) Evaluation of ankle joint function: the use of a scoring scale.
The Foot; 1:15–19.

Content

Type Patient reported outcome
Scale 6 subscales (8 items):

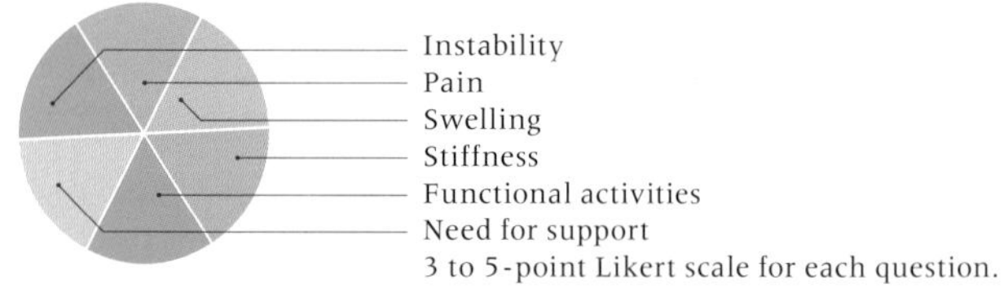

3 to 5-point Likert scale for each question.

Interpretation

Excellent: 90–100 points
Good: 80–89 points
Fair: 60–79 points
Poor: < 60 points
Score normalized to 100.

Validation

Outcomes validated against [1]
- Foot and ankle outcome score

Outcomes validated against [2]
- Radiographic evaluation of ankle joint stability
- Patient assessed ankle function
- St. Pierre ankle score

Patient population tested in	Validity	Reliability	Responsiveness
Patients with anatomical reconstruction of lateral ankle ligaments (39.6 years; 60% male) [1]	+	not tested	not tested
Data identified from another article. Population data not available [2]	+	not tested	+

Validation studies:
[1] Roos EM, Brandsson S, Karlsson J (2001) Validation of the foot and ankle outcome score for ankle ligament reconstruction. Foot Ankle Int; 22:788–794.
[2] Haywood KL, Hargreaves J, Lamb SE (2004) Multi-item outcome measures for lateral ligament injury of the ankle: a structured review. J Eval Clin Pract; 10:339–352.

Methodological evaluation

●●●○○○ (3/6)

		no score	0 points	1 point	points
Validity	Content validity	not tested	not valid	**valid**	1
	Construct validity	not tested	not valid	**valid**	1
	Criterion validity	**not tested**	not valid	valid	-
Reliability	Internal consistency	**not tested**	not consistent	consistent	-
	Reproducibility	**not tested**	not reproducible	reproducible	-
	Responsiveness	not tested	not responsive	**responsive**	1
				Subtotal	**3**

Clinical utility

●●●● (4/4)

	0 points	1 point	2 points	points
Patient friendliness	limited	moderate	**strong**	2
Clinician friendliness	limited	moderate	**strong**	2
			Subtotal	**4**

Total (out of 10) ●●●●●●●○○○ **7**

14. Karlstrom Olerud ankle score (1977)

Source: Karlstrom G, Olerud S (1977) Ipsilateral fracture of the femur and tibia.
J Bone Joint Surg Am; 59:240–243.

Content

Type Clinician based outcome
Scale 7 subscales (7 items):

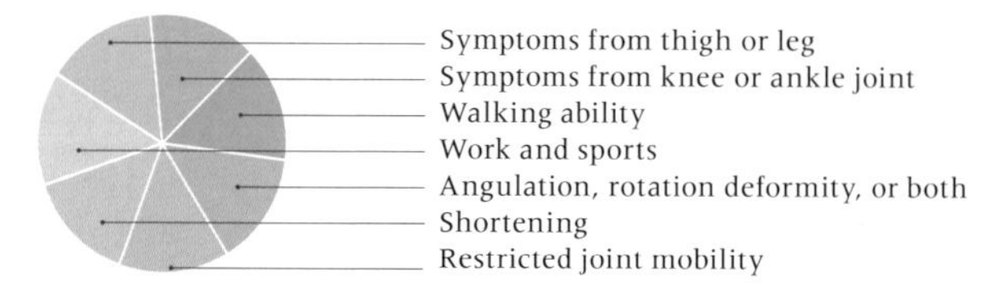

Interpretation

Each rated poor, acceptable, good, or excellent.

Validation

No validation studies were identified.

Patient population tested in	Validity	Reliability	Responsiveness
Not applicable			

Methodological evaluation

○○○○○○ (0/6)

		no score	0 points	1 point	points
Validity	Content validity	not tested	not valid	valid	-
	Construct validity	not tested	not valid	valid	-
	Criterion validity	not tested	not valid	valid	-
Reliability	Internal consistency	not tested	not consistent	consistent	-
	Reproducibility	not tested	not reproducible	reproducible	-
	Responsiveness	not tested	not responsive	responsive	-
				Subtotal	-

Clinical utility

●●○○ (2/4)

	0 points	1 point	2 points	points
Patient friendliness	limited	moderate	strong	2
Clinician friendliness	limited	moderate	strong	0
			Subtotal	2

Total (out of 10) 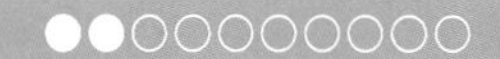 **2**

15. Lesser toe metatarsophalangeal-interphalangeal scale of the American Orthopaedic Foot and Ankle Society (1994)

Source:
Kitaoka HB, Alexander IJ, Adelaar RS, Nunley JA, Myerson MS, Sanders M (1994) Clinical rating systems for the ankle-hindfoot, midfoot, hallux, and lesser toes.
Foot Ankle Int; 15:349-353.

Content

Type Clinician based outcome
Scale 3 subscales (8 items):

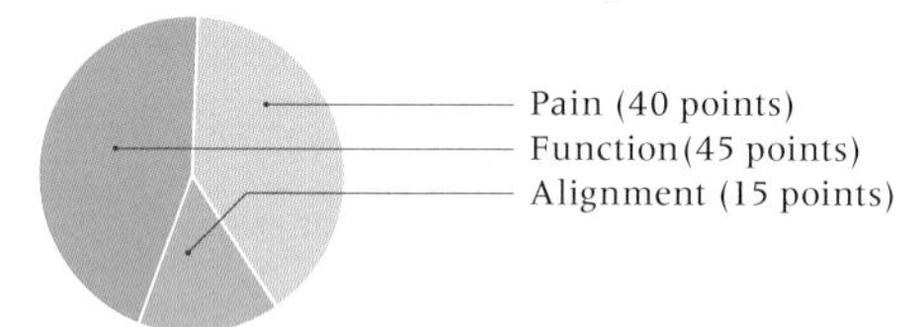

Interpretation

Minimum score: 0 points
Maximum score: 100 points

The higher the score, the higher the function.

Validation

Outcomes validated against

- SF-36

Patient population tested in	Validity	Reliability	Responsiveness
Patients presenting with lesser MTP-IP joint complaints (50 years; 42% male)	+/-	-	not tested

Validation study:

SooHoo NF, Shuler M, Fleming LL (2003) Evaluation of the validity of the AOFAS Clinical Rating Systems by correlation to the SF-36. Foot Ankle Int; 24:50–55.

15. Lesser toe metatarsophalangeal-interphalangeal scale (1994)

Methodological evaluation ●○○○○○ (1/6)

		no score	0 points	1 point	points
Validity	Content validity	not tested	not valid	**valid**	1
Validity	Construct validity	not tested	**not valid**	valid	0
Validity	Criterion validity	**not tested**	not valid	valid	-
Reliability	Internal consistency	**not tested**	not consistent	consistent	-
Reliability	Reproducibility	not tested	**not reproducible**	reproducible	0
	Responsiveness	**not tested**	not responsive	responsive	-
				Subtotal	**1**

Clinical utility ●●●● (4/4)

	0 points	1 point	2 points	points
Patient friendliness	limited	moderate	**strong**	2
Clinician friendliness	limited	moderate	**strong**	2
			Subtotal	**4**

Total (out of 10) ●●●●●○○○○○ **5**

16. Liu ankle score (1995)

Source: Liu SH, Jacobson KE (1995) A new operation for chronic lateral ankle instability.
J Bone Joint Surg Br; 77:55–59.

Content

Type Clinician based outcome
Scale 8 subscales (8 items):

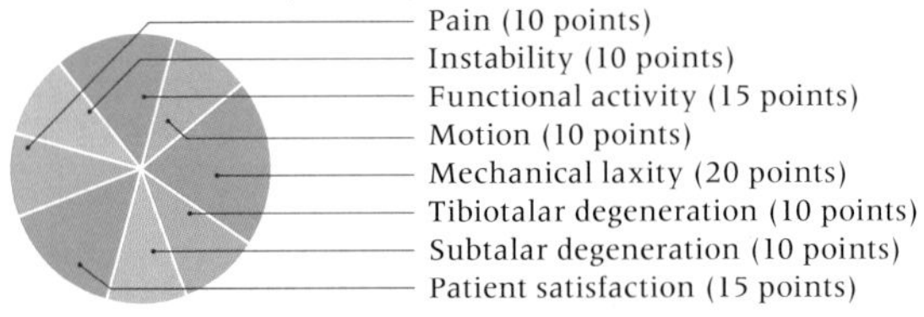

Interpretation

Excellent: 90–100 points
Good: 80–89 points
Fair: 70–79 points
Poor: < 70 points

Validation

No validation studies were identified.

Patient population tested in	Validity	Reliability	Responsiveness
Not applicable			

Methodological evaluation

○○○○○○ (0/6)

		no score	0 points	1 point	points
Validity	Content validity	not tested	not valid	valid	-
	Construct validity	not tested	not valid	valid	-
	Criterion validity	not tested	not valid	valid	-
Reliability	Internal consistency	not tested	not consistent	consistent	-
	Reproducibility	not tested	not reproducible	reproducible	-
	Responsiveness	not tested	not responsive	responsive	-
				Subtotal	-

Clinical utility

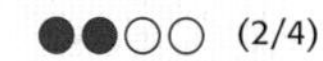

●●○○ (2/4)

	0 points	1 point	2 points	points
Patient friendliness	limited	moderate	strong	2
Clinician friendliness	limited	moderate	strong	0
			Subtotal	2

Total (out of 10)

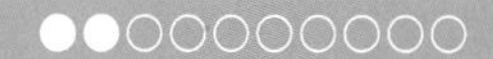

●●○○○○○○○○

2

17. Maryland foot rating score (also known as Painful Foot Center scoring system)* (1993)

Source: Sanders R, Fortin P, DiPasquale T, Walling A (1993) Operative treatment in 120 displaced intraarticular calcaneal fractures. Results using a prognostic computed tomography scan classification. Clin Orthop; (290):87–95.

Content

Type Clinician based outcome
Scale 5 subscales (10 items):

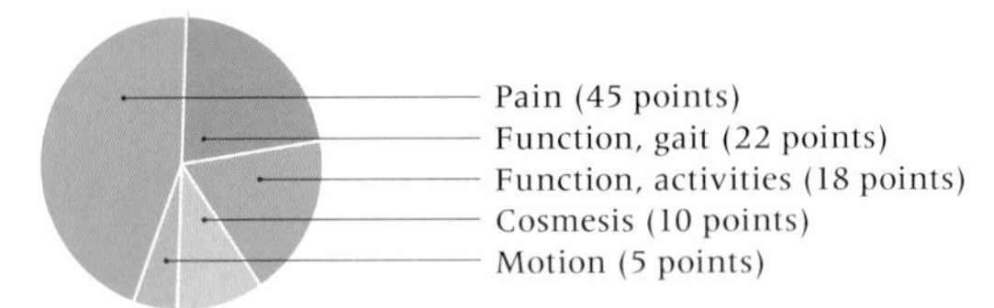

Interpretation
Excellent: 90–100 points
Good: 75–89 points
Fair: 60–74 points
Poor: < 60 points

Validation

No validation studies were identified.

Patient population tested in	Validity	Reliability	Responsiveness
Not applicable			

* *Original information on the development of the Maryland Painful Foot Center Score could not be found.*

17. Maryland foot rating score (also known as Painful Foot Center scoring system (1993)

Methodological evaluation

○○○○○○ (0/6)

		no score	0 points	1 point	points
Validity	Content validity	not tested	not valid	valid	-
	Construct validity	not tested	not valid	valid	-
	Criterion validity	not tested	not valid	valid	-
Reliability	Internal consistency	not tested	not consistent	consistent	-
	Reproducibility	not tested	not reproducible	reproducible	-
	Responsiveness	not tested	not responsive	responsive	-
				Subtotal	-

Clinical utility

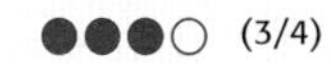
(3/4)

	0 points	1 point	2 points	points
Patient friendliness	limited	moderate	strong	2
Clinician friendliness	limited	moderate	strong	1
			Subtotal	3

Total (out of 10) 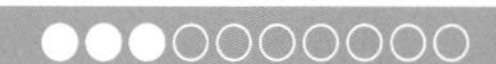 **3**

18. Mazur ankle score (1979)

Source: Mazur JM, Schwartz E, Simon SR (1979) Ankle arthrodesis. Long-term follow-up with gait analysis. J Bone Joint Surg Am; 61:964–975.

Content

Type Clinician based outcome
Scale 3 subscales (12 items):

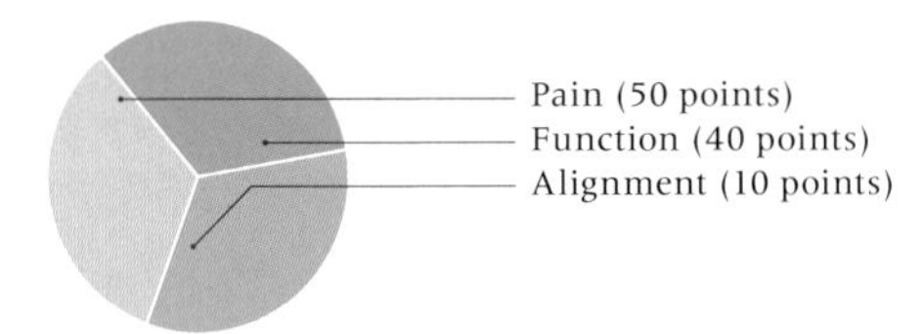

Interpretation

Excellent: 80–100 points
Good: 70–79 points
Fair: 60–69 points
Poor: < 60 points

Validation

No validation studies were identified.

Patient population tested in	Validity	Reliability	Responsiveness
Not applicable			

Methodological evaluation

○○○○○○ (0/6)

		no score	0 points	1 point	points
Validity	Content validity	not tested	not valid	valid	-
	Construct validity	not tested	not valid	valid	-
	Criterion validity	not tested	not valid	valid	-
Reliability	Internal consistency	not tested	not consistent	consistent	-
	Reproducibility	not tested	not reproducible	reproducible	-
	Responsiveness	not tested	not responsive	responsive	-
				Subtotal	-

Clinical utility

●●●● (4/4)

	0 points	1 point	2 points	points
Patient friendliness	limited	moderate	strong	2
Clinician friendliness	limited	moderate	strong	2
			Subtotal	**4**

Total (out of 10) 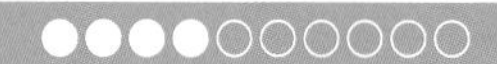 **4**

19. Midfoot scale of the American Orthopaedic Foot and Ankle Society (1994)

Source: Kitaoka HB, Alexander IJ, Adelaar RS, Nunley JA, Myerson MS, Sanders M (1994) Clinical rating systems for the ankle-hindfoot, midfoot, hallux, and lesser toes.
Foot Ankle Int; 15:349–353.

Content

Type Clinician based outcome
Scale 3 subscales (7 items):

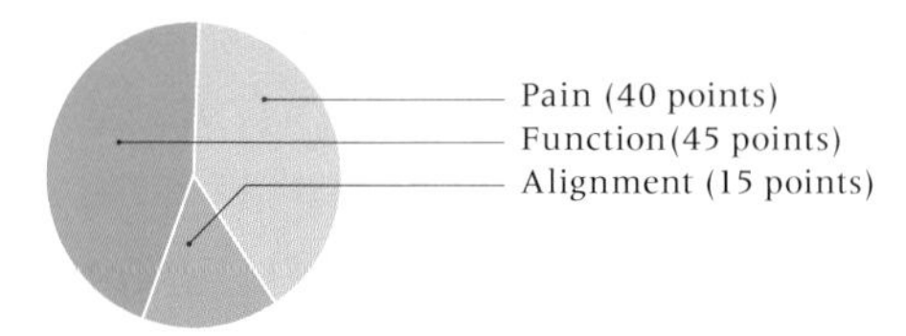

Interpretation

Minimum score: 0 points
Maximum score: 100 points

The higher the score, the higher the function.

Validation

Outcomes validated against

- SF-36

Patient population tested in	Validity	Reliability	Responsiveness
Patients presenting with midfoot complaints (50 years; 42% male)	+/-	-	not tested

Validation study:
SooHoo NF, Shuler M, Fleming LL (2003) Evaluation of the validity of the AOFAS Clinical Rating Systems by correlation to the SF-36. Foot Ankle Int; 24:50–55.

Methodological evaluation

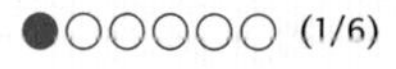
(1/6)

		no score	0 points	1 point	points
Validity	Content validity	not tested	not valid	valid	1
	Construct validity	not tested	not valid	valid	0
	Criterion validity	not tested	not valid	valid	-
Reliability	Internal consistency	not tested	not consistent	consistent	-
	Reproducibility	not tested	not reproducible	reproducible	0
	Responsiveness	not tested	not responsive	responsive	-
				Subtotal	**1**

Clinical utility

(4/4)

	0 points	1 point	2 points	points
Patient friendliness	limited	moderate	strong	2
Clinician friendliness	limited	moderate	strong	2
			Subtotal	**4**

Total (out of 10) 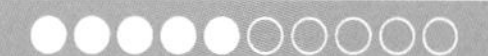 **5**

20. Olerud Molander Ankle score (OMA) (1984)

Source: Olerud C, Molander H (1984) A scoring scale for symptom evaluation after ankle fracture.
Arch Orthop Trauma Surg; 103:190–194.

Content

Type Clinician based outcome
Scale 9 subscales (9 items):

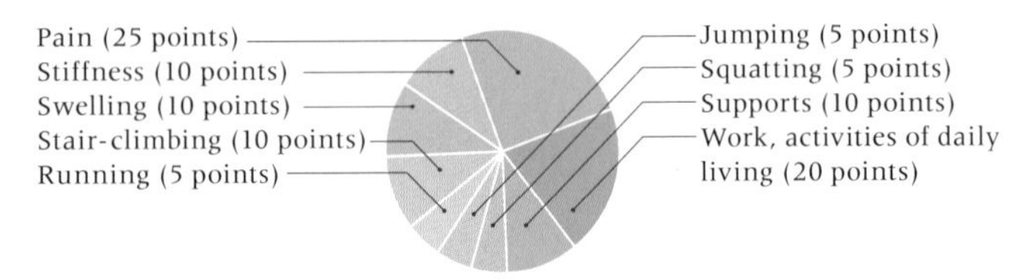

Interpretation

Minimum score: 0 points; maximum score: 100 points
The higher the score, the higher the function.

Validation

Outcomes validated against [1]
- Single subjective question
- Range of motion in loaded dorsal extension
- Presence of osteoarthritis
- Presence of dislocations

Outcomes validated against [2]
- Radiographic evidence of osteoarthritis

Outcomes validated against [3]
- SF-36

Patient population tested in	Validity	Reliability	Responsiveness
Patients with multi-component ankle fractures (age NR; sex NR) [1]	+	not tested	not tested
Arthrodesis of the ankle (30 years; sex NR) [2]	+	not tested	+
B-type ankle fractures (41 years; 50% male) [3]	+	not tested	not tested

Validation studies:

[1] Olerud C, Molander H (1984) A scoring scale for symptom evaluation after ankle fracture. Arch Orthop Trauma Surg; 103:190–194.
[2] Fuchs S, Sandmann C, Skwara A, et al (2003) Quality of life 20 years after arthrodesis of the ankle. A study of adjacent joints. J Bone Joint Surg Br; 85:994–998.
[3] Ponzer S, Nasell H, Bergman B, et al (1999) Functional outcome and quality of life in patients with Type B ankle fractures: a two-year follow-up study. J Orthop Trauma; 13:363–368.

Methodological evaluation ●●○○○○ (2/6)

		no score	0 points	1 point	points
Validity	Content validity	**not tested**	not valid	valid	-
	Construct validity	not tested	not valid	**valid**	1
	Criterion validity	**not tested**	not valid	valid	-
Reliability	Internal consistency	**not tested**	not consistent	consistent	-
	Reproducibility	**not tested**	not reproducible	reproducible	-
	Responsiveness	not tested	not responsive	**responsive**	1
				Subtotal	**2**

Clinical utility ●●○○ (2/4)

	0 points	1 point	2 points	points
Patient friendliness	limited	moderate	**strong**	2
Clinician friendliness	**limited**	moderate	strong	0
			Subtotal	**2**

Total (out of 10) ●●●●○○○○○○ **4**

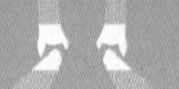

21. Sports Ankle Rating—quality of life measure (2003)

Source: Williams GN, Molloy JM, DeBerardino TM, Arciero RA, Taylor DC (2003) Evaluation of the Sports Ankle Rating System in young, athletic individuals with acute lateral ankle sprains. Foot Ankle Int; 24:274–282.

Content

Type Patient reported outcome
Scale 5 subscales (25 items):

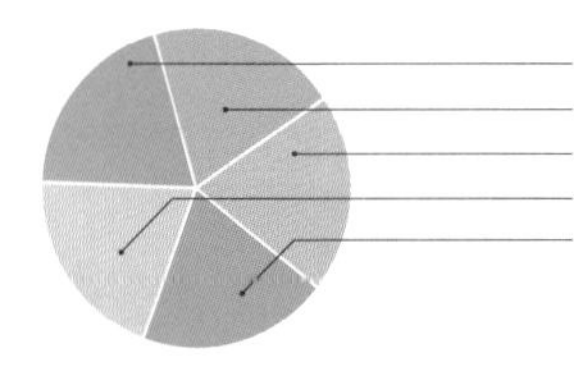

Likert scale for each subscale (0 to 4 points) with 0 points being extreme dysfunction and 4 points being normal function.

Interpretation

Minimum score: 0 points
Maximum score: 20 points

The higher the score, the higher the function.

Validation

Outcomes validated against

- Not applicable—only content validity was assessed.

Patient population tested in	Validity	Reliability	Responsiveness
Patients with grade II lateral ankle sprains (19.7 years; 93% male)	+	not tested	+
Reference group of volunteers who reported "normal" ankle function bilaterally (19.7 years; 80% male)	not tested	+	not tested

Validation study:

Williams GN, Molloy JM, DeBerardino TM, et al (2003) Evaluation of the Sports Ankle Rating System in young, athletic individuals with acute lateral ankle sprains. Foot Ankle Int; 24:274–282.

Methodological evaluation

●●●●○○ (4/6)

		no score	0 points	1 point	points
Validity	Content validity	not tested	not valid	valid	1
	Construct validity	not tested	not valid	valid	-
	Criterion validity	not tested	not valid	valid	-
Reliability	Internal consistency	not tested	not consistent	consistent	1
	Reproducibility	not tested	not reproducible	reproducible	1
	Responsiveness	not tested	not responsive	responsive	1
				Subtotal	**4**

Clinical utility

●●○○ (2/4)

	0 points	1 point	2 points	points
Patient friendliness	limited	moderate	strong	0
Clinician friendliness	limited	moderate	strong	2
			Subtotal	**2**

Total (out of 10) ●●●●●●○○○○ **6**

22. Sports ankle rating system—clinical rating score (2003)

Source: Williams GN, Molloy JM, DeBerardino TM, Arciero RA, Taylor DC (2003) Evaluation of the Sports Ankle Rating System in young, athletic individuals with acute lateral ankle sprains. Foot Ankle Int; 24:274–282.

Content

Type Clinician based outcome
Scale 10 subscales:

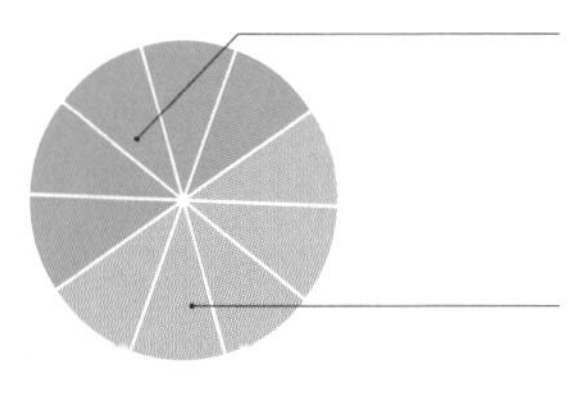

5 patient based subscales:
Pain (8 points)
Swelling (8 points)
Stiffness (8 points)
Giving-way (8 points)
Function (8 points)
5 clinician based subscales:
Gait (10 points)
Motion (10 points)
Strength (10 points)
Stability (10 points)
Postural stability (10 points)
Function (10 points)

Interpretation

Subscale scores can be kept separate or combined
Patient-based subscale score: 0–40 points
Clinician based subscale score: 0–60 points
Combined score: 0–100 points
The higher the score, the higher the function.

Validation

Outcomes validated against

- Not applicable—only content validity was assessed.

Patient population tested in	Validity	Reliability	Responsiveness
Patients with grade II lateral ankle sprains (19.7 years; 93% male)	+	not tested	+
Reference group of volunteers who reported "normal" ankle function bilaterally (19.7 years; 80% male)	not tested	+	not tested

Validation study:

Williams GN, Molloy JM, DeBerardino TM, et al (2003) Evaluation of the Sports Ankle Rating System in young, athletic individuals with acute lateral ankle sprains. Foot Ankle Int; 24:274–282.

22. Sports ankle rating system—clinical rating score (2003)

Methodological evaluation ●●●●○○ (4/6)

		no score	0 points	1 point	points
Validity	Content validity	not tested	not valid	**valid** (selected)	1
Validity	Construct validity	**not tested** (selected)	not valid	valid	-
Validity	Criterion validity	**not tested** (selected)	not valid	valid	-
Reliability	Internal consistency	not tested	not consistent	**consistent** (selected)	1
Reliability	Reproducibility	not tested	not reproducible	**reproducible** (selected)	1
	Responsiveness	not tested	not responsive	**responsive** (selected)	1
				Subtotal	**4**

Clinical utility ●●○○ (2/4)

	0 points	1 point	2 points	points
Patient friendliness	limited	moderate	**strong** (selected)	2
Clinician friendliness	**limited** (selected)	moderate	strong	0
			Subtotal	**2**

Total (out of 10) ●●●●●●○○○○ **6**

23. Sports Ankle Rating–Single Assessment Numeric Evaluation (SANE) (2003)

Source: Williams GN, Molloy JM, DeBerardino TM, Arciero RA, Taylor DC (2003) Evaluation of the Sports Ankle Rating System in young, athletic individuals with acute lateral ankle sprains.
Foot Ankle Int; 24:274–282.

Content

Type Patient reported outcome
Scale

Single question: "On a scale of 0 to 100, how would you rate your ankle function with 100 being normal?"

Interpretation

Minimum score: 0 points
Maximum score: 100 points

The higher the score, the higher the function.

Validation

Outcomes validated against

- Not applicable.

Patient population tested in	Validity	Reliability	Responsiveness
Patients with grade II lateral ankle sprains (19.7 years; 93% male)	not tested	not tested	+
Reference group of volunteers who reported "normal" ankle function bilaterally (19.7 years; 80% male)	not tested	+	not tested

Validation study:

Williams GN, Molloy JM, DeBerardino TM, et al (2003) Evaluation of the Sports Ankle Rating System in young, athletic individuals with acute lateral ankle sprains. Foot Ankle Int; 24:274–282.

23. Sports Ankle Rating—Single Assessment Numeric Evaluation (SANE) (2003)

Methodological evaluation

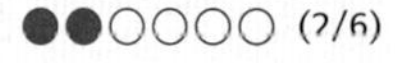
(2/6)

		no score	0 points	1 point	points
Validity	Content validity	not tested	not valid	valid	-
	Construct validity	not tested	not valid	valid	-
	Criterion validity	not tested	not valid	valid	-
Reliability	Internal consistency	not tested	not consistent	consistent	-
	Reproducibility	not tested	not reproducible	reproducible	1
	Responsiveness	not tested	not responsive	responsive	1
				Subtotal	**2**

Clinical utility

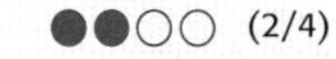
(2/4)

	0 points	1 point	2 points	points
Patient friendliness	limited	moderate	strong	0
Clinician friendliness	limited	moderate	strong	2
			Subtotal	**2**

Total (out of 10) 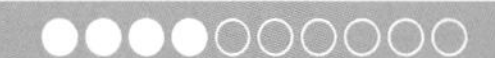 **4**

24. St. Pierre ankle score (1982)

Source: St Pierre R, Allman F Jr, Bassett FH 3rd, Goldner JL, Fleming LL (1982) A review of lateral ankle ligamentous reconstructions. Foot Ankle; 3:114–123.

Content

Type Clinician based outcome
Scale 4 items

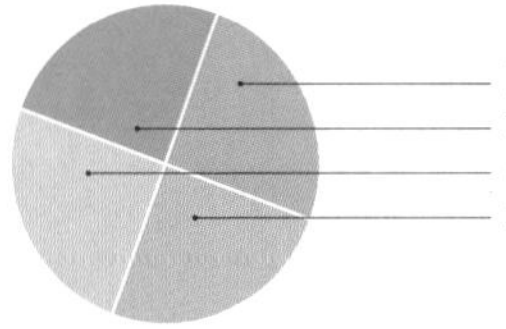

3-point Likert scale for each item (0=excellent, 3=failure).

Interpretation
Excellent: 0 points
Good: 1 points
Fair: 2–6 points
Poor: > 6 points

Validation

No validation studies were identified.

Patient population tested in	Validity	Reliability	Responsiveness
Not applicable			

Methodological evaluation

○○○○○○ (0/6)

		no score	0 points	1 point	points
Validity	Content validity	not tested	not valid	valid	-
	Construct validity	not tested	not valid	valid	-
	Criterion validity	not tested	not valid	valid	-
Reliability	Internal consistency	not tested	not consistent	consistent	-
	Reproducibility	not tested	not reproducible	reproducible	-
	Responsiveness	not tested	not responsive	responsive	-
				Subtotal	-

Clinical utility

 (4/4)

	0 points	1 point	2 points	points
Patient friendliness	limited	moderate	strong	2
Clinician friendliness	limited	moderate	strong	2
			Subtotal	4

Total (out of 10) 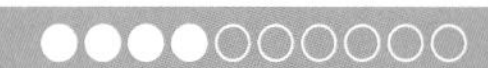 **4**

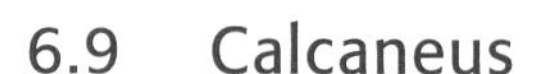

6.9 Calcaneus

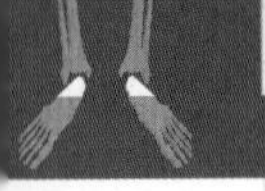

1. Creighton-Nebraska Health Foundation assessment score for fractures of the calcaneus (1996)

Source: Crosby LA, Fitzgibbons TC (1996) Open reduction and internal fixation of type II intra-articular calcaneus fractures. Foot Ankle Int; 17:253–258.

Content

Type Clinician based outcome
Scale 6 subscales (7 items):

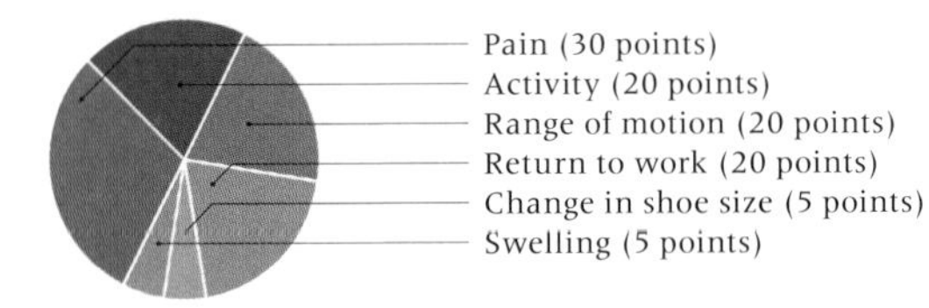

Interpretation

Excellent: 90–100 points
Good: 80–89 points
Fair: 65–79 points
Poor: < 65 points

Validation

No validation studies were identified.

Patient population tested in	Validity	Reliability	Responsiveness
Not applicable			

Methodological evaluation

○○○○○○ (0/6)

		no score	0 points	1 point	points
Validity	Content validity	not tested	not valid	valid	-
	Construct validity	not tested	not valid	valid	-
	Criterion validity	not tested	not valid	valid	-
Reliability	Internal consistency	not tested	not consistent	consistent	-
	Reproducibility	not tested	not reproducible	reproducible	-
	Responsiveness	not tested	not responsive	responsive	-
				Subtotal	-

Clinical utility

●●●○ (3/4)

	0 points	1 point	2 points	points
Patient friendliness	limited	moderate	strong	2
Clinician friendliness	limited	moderate	strong	1
			Subtotal	3

Total (out of 10) 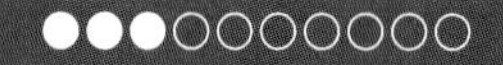 **3**

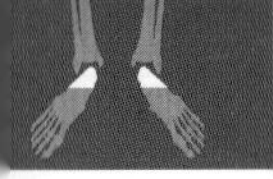

2. Functional outcome assessment of Thordarson (1996)

Source: Thordarson DB, Krieger LE (1996) Operative vs. nonoperative treatment of intra-articular fractures of the calcaneus: a prospective randomized trial.
Foot Ankle Int; 17:2–9.

Content

Type Patient reported outcome
Scale 6 subscales:

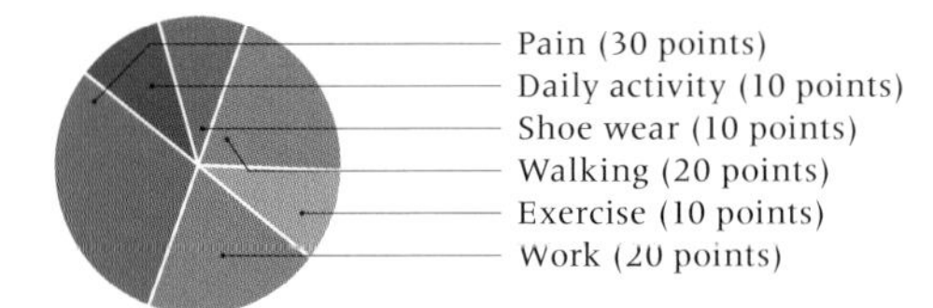

Interpretation

Excellent: 90–100 points
Good: 80–89 points
Fair: 70–79 points
Poor: < 70 points

Validation

Outcomes validated against

- AOFAS ankle-hindfoot scale

Patient population tested in	Validity	Reliability	Responsiveness
Patients with calcaneal fractures: operative group (35 years; 80% male) nonoperative group (36 years; 82% male)	+	not tested	not tested

Validation study:

Thordarson DB, Krieger LE (1996) Operative vs. nonoperative treatment of intra-articular fractures of the calcaneus: a prospective randomized trial. Foot Ankle Int; 17:2–9.

Methodological evaluation

●○○○○○ (1/6)

		no score	0 points	1 point	points
Validity	Content validity	not tested	not valid	valid	-
	Construct validity	not tested	not valid	valid	-
	Criterion validity	not tested	not valid	valid	1
Reliability	Internal consistency	not tested	not consistent	consistent	-
	Reproducibility	not tested	not reproducible	reproducible	-
	Responsiveness	not tested	not responsive	responsive	-
				Subtotal	1

Clinical utility

●●●● (4/4)

	0 points	1 point	2 points	points
Patient friendliness	limited	moderate	strong	2
Clinician friendliness	limited	moderate	strong	2
			Subtotal	4

Total (out of 10) 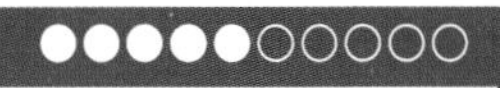 **5**

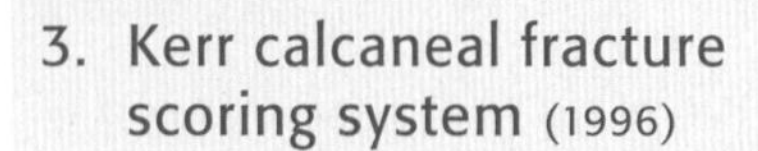

3. Kerr calcaneal fracture scoring system (1996)

Source: Kerr PS, Prothero DL, Atkins RM (1996) Assessing outcome following calcaneal fracture: a rational scoring system. Injury; 27:35–38.

Content

Type Patient reported outcome
Scale 5 subscales:

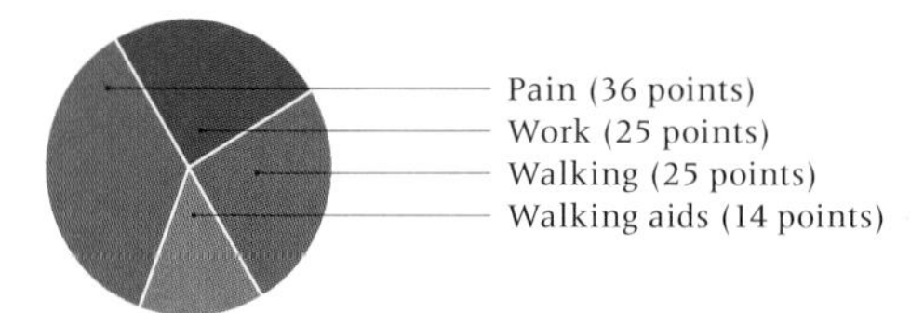

Interpretation

Minimum score: 0 points
Maximum score: 100 points

The higher the score, the higher the function.

Validation

No validation studies were identified.

Patient population tested in	Validity	Reliability	Responsiveness
Patients with intraarticular fractures of the calcaneus (46 years; 72% male)	+	not tested	not tested

Validation study:
Kerr PS, Prothero DL, Atkins RM (1996) Assessing outcome following calcaneal fracture: a rational scoring system. Injury; 27:35–38.

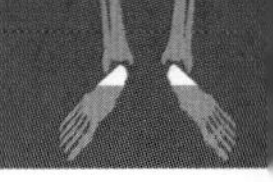

Methodological evaluation

●○○○○○ (1/6)

		no score	0 points	1 point	points
Validity	Content validity	not tested	not valid	**valid**	1
	Construct validity	**not tested**	not valid	valid	-
	Criterion validity	**not tested**	not valid	valid	-
Reliability	Internal consistency	**not tested**	not consistent	consistent	-
	Reproducibility	**not tested**	not reproducible	reproducible	-
	Responsiveness	**not tested**	not responsive	responsive	-
				Subtotal	**1**

Clinical utility

●●●● (4/4)

	0 points	1 point	2 points	points
Patient friendliness	limited	moderate	**strong**	2
Clinician friendliness	limited	moderate	**strong**	2
			Subtotal	**4**

Total (out of 10) 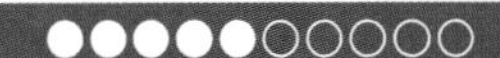 **5**

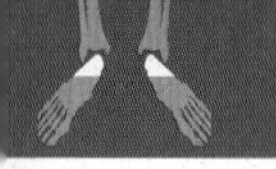

4. Oral analogue scale (1998)

Source: Morin P, Buckley R, Stewart R, Vande Gutche R (1998) Oral analogue scale as an outcome measure after displaced intra-articular calcaneal fractures.
Foot Ankle Int; 19:694–697.

Content

Type Patient reported outcome
Scale

Single question:
"You have suffered a broken heel bone; if the pain from that is a '10' and your normal foot is a '0', where would you put your present (injured) foot in relation to pain and function on the scale of '10' being awful and '0' being normal?"

Interpretation
Minimum score: 0 points
Maximum score: 100 points

The higher the score, the lower the function.

Validation

Outcomes validated against
- VAS for overall result

Patient population tested in	Validity	Reliability	Responsiveness
Patients with displaced intraarticular calcaneal fractures (age NR; % male NR)	+	not tested	not tested

Validation study:
Morin P, Buckley R, Stewart R, et al (1998) Oral analogue scale as an outcome measure after displaced intra-articular calcaneal fractures. Foot Ankle Int; 19:694–697.

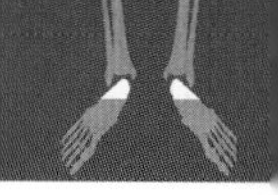

Methodological evaluation

●○○○○○ (1/6)

		no score	0 points	1 point	points
Validity	Content validity	not tested	not valid	valid	-
	Construct validity	not tested	not valid	valid	-
	Criterion validity	not tested	not valid	valid	1
Reliability	Internal consistency	not tested	not consistent	consistent	-
	Reproducibility	not tested	not reproducible	reproducible	-
	Responsiveness	not tested	not responsive	responsive	-
				Subtotal	**1**

Clinical utility

●●●● (4/4)

	0 points	1 point	2 points	points
Patient friendliness	limited	moderate	strong	2
Clinician friendliness	limited	moderate	strong	2
			Subtotal	**4**

Total (out of 10) 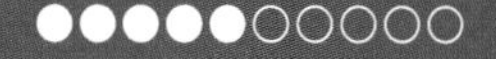 **5**

5. Paley scoring system (1993)

Source: Paley D, Hall H (1993) Intra-articular fractures of the calcaneus. A critical analysis of results and prognostic factors. J Bone Joint Surg Am; 75:342–354.

Content

Type Clinician based outcome
Scale 8 subscales (9 items):

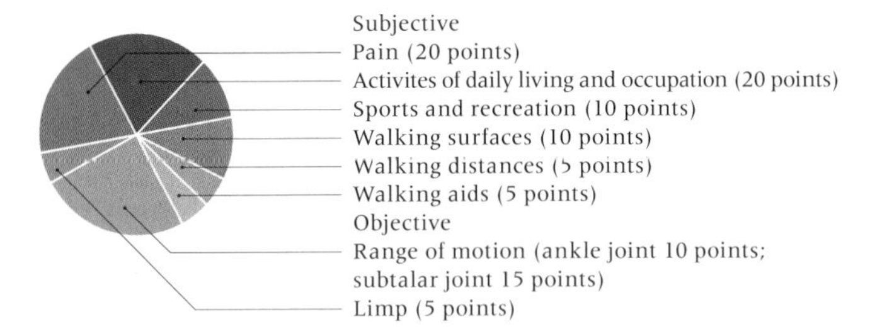

Interpretation
Excellent: 90–100 points
Good: 72–89 points
Fair: 41–71 points
Poor: < 41 points

Validation

No validation studies were identified.

Patient population tested in	Validity	Reliability	Responsiveness
Not applicable			

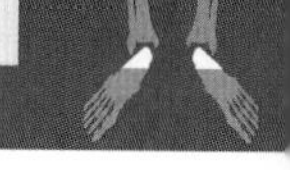

Methodological evaluation ○○○○○○ (0/6)

		no score	0 points	1 point	points
Validity	Content validity	not tested	not valid	valid	-
	Construct validity	not tested	not valid	valid	-
	Criterion validity	not tested	not valid	valid	-
Reliability	Internal consistency	not tested	not consistent	consistent	-
	Reproducibility	not tested	not reproducible	reproducible	-
	Responsiveness	not tested	not responsive	responsive	-
				Subtotal	-

Clinical utility ●●○○ (2/4)

	0 points	1 point	2 points	points
Patient friendliness	limited	moderate	strong	2
Clinician friendliness	limited	moderate	strong	0
			Subtotal	2

Total (out of 10) 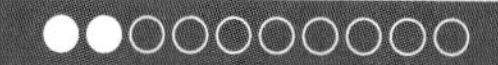 **2**

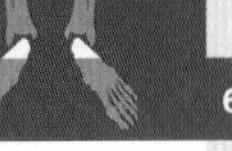

6. Visual analog scale of Hildebrand (1996)

Source: Hildebrand KA, Buckley RE, Mohtadi NG (1996) Functional outcome measures after displaced intra-articular calcaneal fractures. J Bone Joint Surg Br; 78:119–123.

Content

Type Clinician based outcome
Scale 3 subscales (16 items):

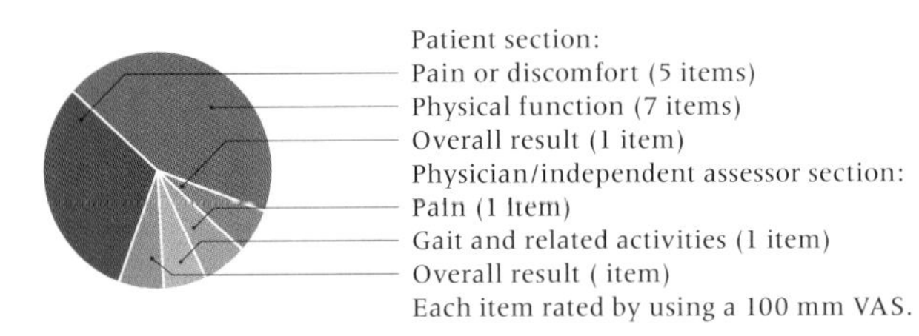

Interpretation

Mean of all VAS scores gives total score

Minimum: 0 points
Maximum: 100 points

Validation

Outcomes validated against

- Modified Rowe score
- McGill Pain Questionnaire
- SF-36

Patient population tested in	Validity	Reliability	Responsiveness
Patients with intraarticular fractures of the posterior facet of the calcaneus (43 years; 100% male)	+	+	not tested

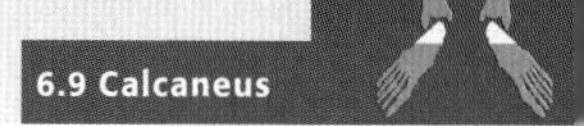

Methodological evaluation

●●○○○○ (2/6)

		no score	0 points	1 point	points
Validity	Content validity	**not tested**	not valid	valid	-
	Construct validity	not tested	not valid	**valid**	1
	Criterion validity	**not tested**	not valid	valid	-
Reliability	Internal consistency	**not tested**	not consistent	consistent	-
	Reproducibility	not tested	not reproducible	**reproducible**	1
	Responsiveness	**not tested**	not responsive	responsive	-
				Subtotal	2

Clinical utility

●●●● (4/4)

	0 points	1 point	2 points	points
Patient friendliness	limited	moderate	**strong**	2
Clinician friendliness	limited	moderate	**strong**	2
			Subtotal	4

Total (out of 10)

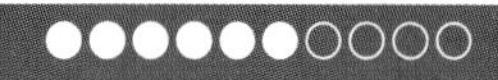

6

7 Recommendations

1 Evaluating outcomes instruments: choosing the right one

Outcome instruments are designed to provide musculoskeletal clinicians and researchers the data necessary for self-improvement and critical evaluation. For the practicing clinician, evaluating the results of one's own intervention and assessing the results reported by others in the literature is often as important as understanding the technique itself. For clinicans, epidemiologists, and clinical researchers, outcomes measurements are essential to advancing education and developing new techniques.

This book is designed to ease the burden of evaluating the appropriate use of a specific outcomes instrument in the reported literature. As an easy-to-read handbook, it will enable readers to gain a fuller appreciation of the context in which a particular outcomes instrument was chosen by an author and its relationship to the outcomes measured. Armed with that information, clinicians will better be able to critically evaluate the reported literature.

This book also reviews two major divisions of outcomes measures and instruments: clinician based outcomes (CBO) and patient reported outcomes (PRO). As there is a strong movement in clinical trials to use PROs when assessing the effects of interventions used to arrest or reverse a potential decline in patient function [1], increased attention is being given to patients' preferences, wishes, and evaluation of their health care outcomes [2].

There has been considerable debate in the musculoskeletal literature as to whether both PROs and CBOs (eg, knee stability, range of motion, x-ray findings, etc.) should both be used given the possibility of disagreement between the two . In the end, one needs to balance the purpose of the study, the stated hypotheses, and the expected effects of a specific intervention.
Given the importance of patients' perceptions, we recommend the use of the most relevant disease-specific PRO when evaluating

the results of a given treatment. The use of additional CBOs and generic PROs to supplement these measures may depend on the overall burden on both the patient and the staff when selecting a battery of outcomes instruments. There are several instruments presented in this handbook that received a high score by adhering to the methodological and clinical utility concepts discussed in chapter 3. However, the score alone should not dictate whether one selects one outcomes measure over another. Before selecting an instrument, it is imperative to ensure that it is appropriate for the population being evaluated. You must make certain that the content of the instrument is appropriate and that the testing was done in a population similar to the one of interest.

Questions to consider when evaluating and choosing the most appropriate outcomes instruments for a given situation are listed in checklist 1.

Checklist 1: choosing, evaluating, and developing the methodological and clinical utility concepts an outcome instrument.*

1	**Is the instrument internally consistent?**	√
2	**Is the instrument reproducible?**	√
3	**Does the instrument demonstrate criterion validity?**	√
4	**Does the instrument demonstrate construct validity?**	√
5	**Does the instrument demonstrate content validity?**	√
6	**Does the instrument detect changes over time that matter to patients?**	√
7	**Will this instrument be deemed acceptable by patients?**	√
8	**Is this instrument feasible to administer clinically?**	√

* These concepts should also be considered and tested when developing an instrument (see next section).

2 Developing outcomes instruments: points to consider

This handbook represents our effort to evaluate nearly 150 musculoskeletal outcomes instruments in a consistent and effective manner. Recognizing that circumstances, populations and environments may vary widely, it is clear that few instruments may be generically applied in all clinical situations. If you are in a setting with a unique population and there are no instruments that are appropriate for your patient or study population, then the development of a new instrument is appropriate. For example, if you are measuring the effectiveness of the Locking Compression Plate (LCP) in the treatment of tibial plateau fractures among young males, you may not be able to find an appropriate instrument, despite there being more than 20 common knee instruments reported in the literature. Such an example, and others like this, may require the development of a new instrument.

Developing a new outcomes instrument is no easy endeavor and this handbook alone will not provide a recipe for doing so. However, it will be a useful resource in getting you started and monitoring your progress. You will need other resources and a team of experts to be successful. Below are our 10 "lessons learned" from evaluating nearly 150 musculoskeletal outcomes instruments that should be considered when developing a new instrument (see checklist 2).

1. Many instruments are named after the author who developed it. Instruments should be given a name that accurately describes their content. Multiple names for the same instrument should be avoided. If an instrument has been revised or abbreviated, it should be indicated in the title.

2. Though the methodological concepts of validity and reliability are well recognized, few developers take into account the important *clinical utility* concepts that we have defined as "patient friendliness" and "clinician friendliness". Though these are not scientific per se, they should be included in the process of content development.

3. Few instruments have gone through a formal process of developing the content or if they have, this process has not been described. Content development for a new instrument is best accomplished by a team of experts to include clinicians, methodologists, and patients. A recommended checklist for content development is provided in checklist 3.

4. Many instruments have not gone through validity and reliability testing. For those that have, often only some concepts are evaluated while others are left untested. When testing an instrument, consider the items in checklist 1. This should be done after the content has been established.

5. While validity and reliability testing may have been performed in conjunction with the development of a new instrument, there are few instruments that are tested by other authors in different patient populations, which limits the instrument's generalizeability. Consider testing a new instrument in more than one type of population.

6. It was at times difficult to identify the source of an instrument (eg, manual or published article) that provided a full description of its purpose, the population for which it was designed, the populations on which it has been tested, and the intended use of the data collected. Consider developing a manual that provides a full description of the instrument's purpose and the populations in which it was designed and tested.

7. A complete version of the instrument was often difficult to find. Such a resource should be made available even if it is for a cost.

8. The scoring of each method was at times difficult to determine. Rarely was there a description of how missing data were handled. Instructions should be made available and clear enough to ensure standard administration and scoring of the method.

9. Once developed, few instruments appeared to go through refinement or improvements. Few, if any, measures are perfect when they are first published and many leading scales in other medical specialties have undergone revisions.

10. Leadership, communication, and oversight by collaborative teams in the development of musculoskeletal outcomes instruments may improve the quality and standardization of both new and existing instruments.

Checklist 2: for developing a new musculoskeletal outcomes instrument.

1	Give the instrument a name that accurately describes its content.	√
2	Develop the content of the instrument by using a team of clinicians, methodologists, and patients (see checklist 3).	√
3	Ensure the clinical utility of the instrument by considering the patient and staff burden of completing, managing, and analyzing the instrument.	√
4	Subject the instrument to the complete battery of validity, reliability and responsiveness testing if appropriate (see checklist 1).	√
5	Encourage other authors to test your instrument in different patient populations.	√
6	Develop a manual and publish an article that provides a full description of the instrument's purpose and the populations in which it was designed and tested.	√
7	Make this manual easily available to the public at a cost if necessary to ensure its frequency and appropriateness of use.	√
8	Provide a clear and concise description of how the instrument is scored and interpreted.	√
9	Be willing to accept criticism and advice from other users and use that information to further refine and improve the instrument.	√
10	Participate in the standardization of outcomes through collaboration and communication with other musculoskeletal outcome instrument developers.	√

Checklist 3: for developing the content of a new musculoskeletal outcomes instrument.

1	Establish a team of individuals that include clinicians, methodologists, and patients.	√
2	Specify the purpose and aims of developing this new instrument.	√
3	Identify all the activities, behaviors, and symptoms that are important to this patient population.	√
4	Consider the potential patient and staff burden in completing or administering the instrument.	√
5	Develop the initial set of questions. Take the necessary time to review and revise.	√
6	Perform a pilot test by administering these questions to a small sample of patients representative of the population of interest. Revise the questions as necessary.	√
7	Field test the existing instrument in a larger sample of patients representative of the population of interest. Revise the questions as necessary.	√
8	Use the appropriate psychometric scaling methods to arrive at the optimal number and type of sub-scales and questions*.	√
9	Establish the subscales and questions for the final version of the instrument.	√

* This topic is beyond the scope of this book.

To help overcome the current limitations in the development of musculoskeletal outcomes and to provide leadership in this area, the AO Foundation with its divsion "AO Clinical Investigation and Documentation" (AOCID) is committed to providing assistance in these areas. AOCID, headquartered in Davos, Switzerland, will provide a board of physicians and epidemiologists whose role is to review, give advice, and make global recommendations in the use and development of musculoskeletal outcomes instruments. To access this service visit AOCID on the AO Foundation's website: http://www.aofoundation.org.

3 References

[1] Roos, E (2000) Rigorous statistical reliability, validity, and responsiveness testing of the Cincinnati Knee Rating System in 350 subjects with uninjured, injured, or anterior cruciate ligament-reconstructed knee. Am J Sports Med; 28:436–438.
[2] Till JE, Sutherland HJ, Meslin EM (1992) Is there a role for preference assessments in research on quality of life in oncology? Qual Life Res; 1:31–40.

8 Appendix: identifying and evaluating musculoskeletal outcomes instruments

1 Explanation of search strategy

Our intent was to identify joint-specific musculoskeletal patient-reported and clinician based outcomes instruments reported in the literature. We intended to identify the most commonly used instruments. Therefore; if an instrument had a history of consistent use then it was included. We limited our search to instruments that were completed by the patient, by the clinician if it included more than one clinical measure (ie, combination of function, range of motion, strength, and activites of daily living), or by both the patient and clinician. Outcomes instruments that reported a single measure or score based on one physiologic outcome (ie, range of motion or radiological findings) were not included in this book.

We included the three most commonly reported generic health-related quality of life instruments in the musculoskeletal literature: the short form 36 health survey questionnaire (SF-36), the Nottingham Health Profile (NHP), and the Musculoskeletal Functional Assessment (MFA).

Our approach to identifying musculoskeletal outcomes instruments was detailed and exhaustive. We began our process by searching all of MEDLINE® with a relatively generic search code to identify as many possible references in the literature that may contain a musculoskeletal outcomes instrument. We placed no limits on the date of publication because some outcomes instruments developed several decades ago are still being used today. From a large list of initial references, additional outcomes instruments were identified by reviewing the text and bibliographies of full-text articles.

Additional instruments were identified by using generic Internet search engines (ie, Google™). A list of outcomes instruments per body area was compiled and built upon throughout the search process. From this list, we first sought to locate the original article, then *all* studies in the literature that evaluated the instruments reproducibility, validity (content, criterion, and construct), responsiveness, or internal consistency. For some, such evaluations were not reported in the literature. For others, there may have been one to several studies reported. The process was lengthy but in the end we felt confident that we were able to identify the majority of the most common musculoskeletal patient reported outcomes (PRO) and clinical based outcomes (CBO) in the literature. Each instrument was reviewed and summarized with respect to four major categories: *content, methodological evaluation, clinical utility,* and *scoring.*

2 Summary of outcomes instrument "content"

Purpose

The purpose of the instrument *content* is to give the user a quick reference for understanding what the instrument is attempting to measure and how the original author(s) recommends it be quantified and interpreted.

Method

We divided each instrument into five major *content* areas:

Name	Most commonly used name in the literature. In some instances, an instrument was referred to by more than one name – if the pattern was consistent, both were included.
References	The original article and subsequent articles that evaluated the instrument's validity, reliability, responsiveness, and internal consistency are provided in the bibliography.
Type	Three types were included: clinician based, patient reported or a combination of clinician and patient based instruments.

Scale The scales and subscales used to evaluate patient status (ie, pain, gait, ADLs) and their respective scoring systems (if applicable).

Interpretation How the original author intended the results of the scales and/or subscales to be interpreted. In some cases, the higher the score the higher the function. In other cases, the higher the score the lower the function. Furthermore, some authors chose to categorize scores into qualitative ratings such as "poor", "fair", "good", and "excellent".

3 Summary of outcomes instrument "methodological evaluation"

Purpose

The purpose of the instrument's *methodological evaluation* is to give the user a quick-reference to what populations the instruments were evaluated in and how the instruments performed when subject to formal evaluation in the literature.

Method

The concepts defined in chapter 3 were the bases of this evaluation. For some instruments, there was no record of evaluation. For those that were subject to evaluation, all studies reporting results were referenced. We report results based on the interpretation of the author(s) who evaluated the instrument's *validity (content, criterion, and construct)*, *reproducibility*, *internal consistency*, and *responsiveness*.

Validity	We reported the characteristics of the populations the instruments were evaluated in (injury or treatment, mean age, and gender distribution), the outcomes the instruments were evaluated against, and whether the instruments were found to be valid or invalid.
Reliability*	We reported the characteristics of the populations the instruments were evaluated in (injury or treatment, mean age, and gender distribution), and whether the instruments were found to be reliable or not reliable.
Responsiveness	We reported the characteristics of the populations the instruments were evaluated in (injury or treatment, mean age, and gender distribution), and whether the instruments were found to be responsive or not responsive.

* The concept of reliability is made up of reproducibility and internal consistency (see chapter 3).

4 Summary of outcomes instrument "clinical utility" evaluation

Purpose

The purpose of the instrument's *clinical utility* is to give the user a quick-reference of the relative patient and staff burden imposed by using the instrument.

Method

While an instrument may contain the appropriate content and demonstrate adequate methods, it may be difficult to administer. Therefore, we reported results with respect to each instrument's *patient friendliness* and *clinician friendliness.*

Patient friendliness	After reviewing the content of each instrument, we determined whether or not the instrument would be deemed acceptable by patients with respect to patient burden.
Clinician friendliness	After reviewing the content of each instrument, we determined whether or not the instrument would be feasible to administer clinically with respect to staff burden.

5 Summary of instrument total score

Purpose

The purpose of the instrument total *score* is to summarize the concepts from the *methodological evaluation* and the *clinical utility* of the instrument to give the reader a relative measure with which to compare each instrument.

Method

All instruments were subject to a formal scoring system designed by us. Eight questions reflecting the *methodological evaluation* and *clinical utility* were designed, Table. Results for the methodological evaluation (*internal consistency, reliability, validities, and responsiveness*) were based on the published interpretation of the authors who evaluated the instruments. Results for clinical utility (*patient friendliness and clinician friendliness*) were based on our judgment.

Conceivably, an instrument could receive a score between 0 to 10 points; six possible points corresponding to the *methodological evaluation* and four possible points corresponding to the *clinical utility evaluation*. Each methodological concept could receive "no points", "0 points", or "1 point" corresponding to whether the concept was found "not tested", "unfavorable" (eg, not valid), or "favorable" (eg, valid), respectively. Each clinical utility concept could receive "0 points", "1 point", or "2 points" corresponding to whether the concept was found "limited", "moderate", or "strong", respectively.

6 Justification for the scoring system

We did not critically appraise the reported findings from articles that evaluated the six methodological concepts (*internal consistency, reliability, criterion validity, construct validity, content validity, and responsiveness*). In other words, we did not evaluate the methods used or the author's interpretation of the results. This process would have been very complicated and subject to personal opinion and interpretation. Instead, we chose to rely on the interpretation of the author(s) who performed the evaluation.

For internal *consistency, reliability, criterion and construct validity,* and *responsiveness,* we evaluated whether or not the authors formally tested the concept and made a specific claim. For those that did, we reported the authors' interpretation of the results. If a claim was not made, other methods of interpreting the authors' findings were employed as seen in the Figure. In cases of multiple evaluation studies with conflicting results, we gave the instrument a positive result if the majority (eg, 2 out of 3) were favorable. If there were two studies that disagreed, we gave the instrument a neutral result (0 points). We did not determine the reason for the discrepancy or judge the relative merits of the studies. Disagreements happened rarely.

When an instrument's *responsiveness* was compared to other instruments for a specific condition (eg, TKA), and found to have the lowest responsiveness among the group of instruments and therefore not favored by the authors, we declared it "not responsive" (0 points).

Since *content and face validity* (distinction made in chapter 3) were rarely evaluated separately in the musculoskeletal literature, and in fact, were often used interchangeably, we decided to combine them as one form of validity that assesses the content of the instrument. Therefore, if the authors described a process by which a team of "experts" corroborated on the content of the instrument (believed to be important components of a disease for which the instrument was created), it received a point (positive result). Content determined by "experts" alone is arguably not sufficient for assessing face validity. Rather, it is often recommended that patients be involved in the process. There were few cases where patients were ever involved; however, dozens of cases where a team of "experts" developed the questionnaire. Given the continuous nature of this type of validity, a point was given in either case. Furthermore, if statistical testing was performed (eg, regression) that included several questions about various health issues and the questions remaining were those determined by their ability to predict a specific outcome (ie, content validity), it received a point.

Correlation coefficients for both reliability and validity were not interpreted or reported in this handbook. There is debate as to the minimal standards for reliability and validity coefficients. It can also be argued that absolute minimal acceptable coefficients are not meaningful, since larger sample sizes for a study allow for more measurement error in an instrument. Hence, we did not rely on them for evaluating these instruments. However, individual coefficients for all measures can be identified in the articles from the reference lists we have provided.

It is preferable to directly assess patient and staff views about a new questionnaire when evaluating its *patient friendliness* and *clinician friendliness*. Some argue that this process should occur during the pre-testing phase of an instrument development, prior to formal tests for reliability and validity. Given little evidence in the musculoskeletal literature of this being done, we applied our clinical and research experience in evaluating these concepts.

Methodological and clinical utility concepts, corresponding questions, and criteria for scoring.

Concept	Question	Criteria
Content validity	Does the author report the outcome demonstrates content validity?	A statement by the author and evidence that the content was developed by a team of professionals or through statistical modeling.
Construct validity*	Does the author report the outcome demonstrates construct validity?	A statement by the author and evidence that the instrument was validated against a generic instrument or correlated with hypothesized subscales from another instrument.
Criterion validity*	Does the author report the outcome demonstrates criterion validity?	A statement by the author and evidence that the instrument was validated against a "gold standard" instrument or predictive of a future outcome.
Internal consistency*	Does the author report the outcome to be internally consistent?	A statement by the author and evidence that it was evaluated by statistical modeling.
Reproducibility*	Does the author report the outcome to be reproducible?	A statement by the author and evidence that it was formally tested.
Responsiveness*	Does the author report the outcome detects changes over time that matter to patients?	A statement by the author and evidence that it was formally tested.

* These concepts should only be considered favorable or unfavorable in the patient populations they were evaluated in and instruments or measures they were validated against.

Patient friendliness	Will this outcome be deemed acceptable by patients?	The following questions were considered: • Can the instrument be completed in a relatively short amount of time? • Are the questions clear, concise, and easy to understand? • Will patients be uncomfortable answering the questions?
Clinician friendliness	Is this outcome feasible to administer clinically?	The following questions were considered: • Is this instrument completed by the staff or self administered? • What is the staff effort and cost in administering, recording, and analyzing? • How much time is required to train the staff in administering the instrument?

Decision trees for determining how to score each instrument with respect to the six methodological concepts.

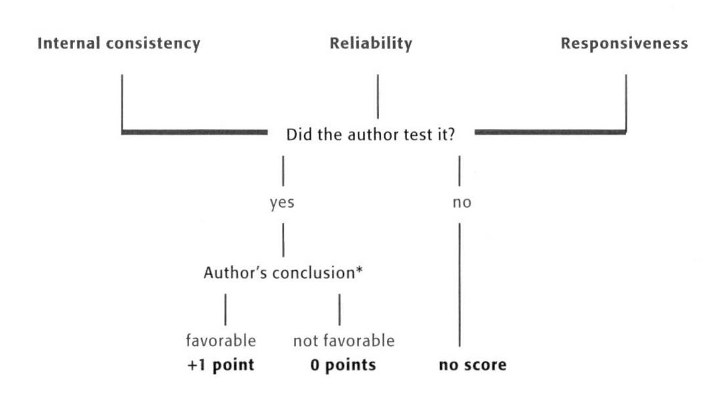

* Based on criteria set forth in the methodological concepts table.

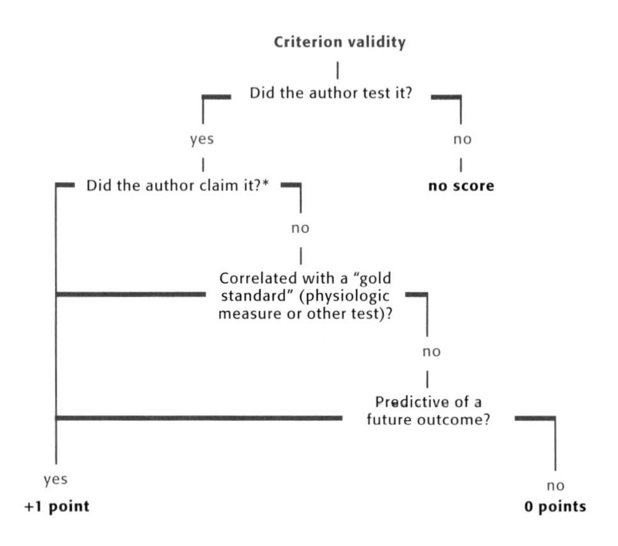
Criterion validity
Did the author test it?
yes
no
Did the author claim it?*
no score
no
Correlated with a "gold standard" (physiologic measure or other test)?
no
Predictive of a future outcome?
yes
+1 point
no
0 points

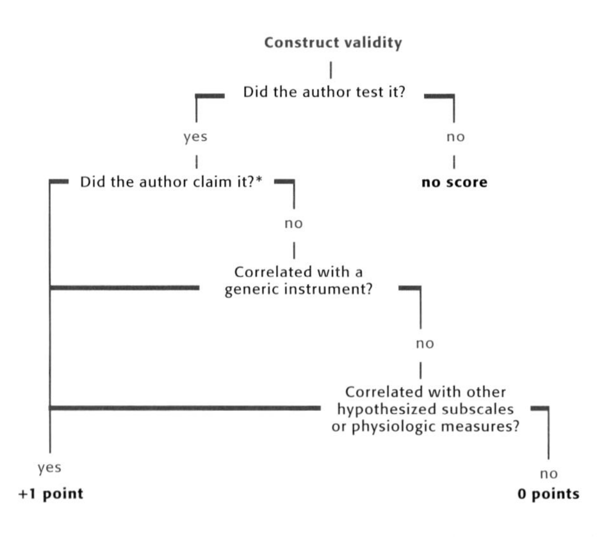
Construct validity
Did the author test it?
yes
no
Did the author claim it?*
no score
no
Correlated with a generic instrument?
no
Correlated with other hypothesized subscales or physiologic measures?
yes
+1 point
no
0 points

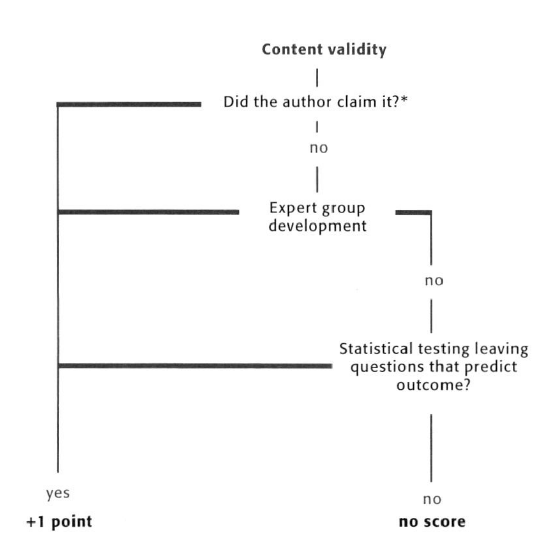

* Based on criteria set forth in the methodological concepts table.

9 List of abbreviations

AAOS	American Association of Orthopaedic Surgeons
AC	Acromioclavicular
ACL	Anterior cruciate ligament
ADL	Activities of daily living
AIMS	Arthritis Impact Measure Scales
AJFAT	Ankle Joint Functional Assessment Tool
AKS	American Knee Society score
AOFAS	The American Orthopaedic Foot and Ankle Society
AOS	Ankle Osteoarthritis Scale
ASES	American Shoulder and Elbow Society scoring system
CBO	Clinician based outcome
COPM	Canadian Occupational Performance Measure
CRS	Cincinnati Knee Rating System
DASH	Disabilities of the Arm Shoulder and Hand questionnaire
EFA	Elbow Functional Assessment scale
FAOS	Foot and Ankle Outcome Score
FFI	Foot Function Index
FHSQ	Foot Health Status Questionnaire
FLEX-SF	Flexilevel scale of Shoulder Function
FRS	Functional Recovery Score
HAQ	Health Assessment Questionnaire (Stanford)
HFI	Hand Functional Index
HOOS	Hip disability and Osteoarthritis Outcome Score
HSS	Hospital for Special Surgery
IKDC	International Knee Documentation Committee knee scoring system

IM	Intramedullary
IP	Interphalangeal
KOOS	Knee Injury and Osteoarthritis Outcome Score
LAI	Lequesne - Algofunctional index
LEFS	Lower Extremity Functional Scale
LEM	Lower Extremity Measure
MACTAR	McMaster-Toronto Arthritis questionnaire
MHQ	Michigan Hand Questionnaire outcome
MPI	Mayo elbow Performance Index
MTP	Metatarsophalangeal
NHP	Nottingham Health Profile
NR	Not reported
NYOH	New York Orthopaedic Hospital
OA	Osteoarthritis
OAS	Oral Analogue Scale
OKS	Oxford Knee Score
OMA	Olerud Molander Ankle score
OSS	Oxford Shoulder Scale
PASI	Patient Specific Index
PFC	Painful Foot Center scoring system
PRO	Patient reported outcome
PREE	Patient Rated Elbow Evaluation
PRWE	Patient Rated Wrist Evaluation
QoL	Quality of life
RAOS	Rheumatoid and Arthritis Outcome Score
RC-QOL	Rotator Cuff Quality of Life measure

ROM	Range of motion
SANE	Single Assessment Numeric Evaluation
SDQ	Shoulder Disability Questionnaire
SF-12	Short form 12 health survey questionnaire
SF-36	Short form 36 health survey questionnaire
SIP	Sickness Impact Profile
SODA	Sequential Occupational Dexterity Assessment
SPADI	Shoulder Pain and Disability Index
SSRS	Subjective Shoulder Rating System
SST	Simple Shoulder Test
THA	Total hip arthroplasty
TKA	Total knee arthroplasty
VAS	Visual analog scale
VRS	Verbal rating system
WOMAC	Western Ontario McMaster University Osteoarthritis index
WOOS	Western Ontario Osteoarthritis of the Shoulder index
WORC	Western Ontario Rotator Cuff

10 Glossary and definitions

Acceptability The extent to which an outcomes instrument is acceptable to patients.

Clinical utility A measure of how "friendly" an outcome is for patients to complete and for clinicians to administer.

Clinician based outcomes (CBO) These measures combine physiologic, surgeon-based, and some patient reported outcomes. Clinician based outcomes are often given a continuous numerical score that is summarized into categorical ratings of "excellent, good, fair, or poor". These ratings can lead to differing conclusions due the to lack of standardized definitions of rating terms.

Clinician friendliness Also known as feasibility. The extent to which the instrument considers the burden on staff and researchers who administer, collect, and process the information with respect to time, cost, and necessary training.

Construct validity A more quantitative form of assessing validity that is evaluated by comparing the relationship of a construct within an instrument (eg, pain) against a hypothesized similar construct within another instrument (eg, SF-36 physical function) or a similar measure (eg, pain medication use).

Content The components of an instrument that include its type (clinician based or patient reported), its scale (the questions that make up the instrument) and the interpretation of the instrument's scoring.

Content validity A form of validity that examines the extent to which the domain of interest is comprehensively sampled by the items, or questions, in the instrument.

Criterion validity A from of validity that considers whether an instrument correlates highly with a "gold standard" measure of the same theme.

Disease specific outcomes measure A measure that attempts to quantify function following the disease, injury or treatment of a specific joint or body part (see joint-specific outcomes measure).

Face validity A form of validity that examines whether an instrument appears to be measuring what it is intended to measure.

Feasibility The extent to which an instrument is feasible to administer clinically with respect to staff burden.

Health-related quality of life Perceived well-being that includes the patient's physical, mental and social health.

Internal consistency A form of reliability that measures how homogenous or consistent the questions in an instrument's scale are and to what extent they are measuring the same thing.

Inter-observer reproducibility The ability of the measure to produce the same results with repeat assessment by different observers rating the same experience.

Intra-observer reproducibility The ability of the measure to produce the same results with repeat assessment by the same observer when no important dimension of health has changed.

Joint-specific outcomes measure A measure that attempts to quantify function following the disease, injury, or treatment of a specific joint or body part (see disease specific outcome measure).

Likert scale An outcomes scale that asks respondents of questionnaires to choose from several responses in a range such as „strongly agree“ to "strongly disagree" or "excellent" to "failure". Each response receives a number rating from 1–5. The 5-point Likert scale is the most common.

Methodology The systematic evaluation of the properties inherent in an outcomes measure. In this context, it refers to the evaluation of an outcome's validity, reliability and responsiveness.

Ordinal scale A scale that recognizes measurement order in the sense that one value is relatively higher or better than another. However, the intervals between values are not necessarily equal or important. An example of an ordinal scale frequently used in orthopedic surgery is the "Excellent, Good, Fair, Poor" scale.

Outcomes measure A measure that adequately quantifies the success (or failure) of a treatment intervention.

Outcomes research The discipline that describes, interprets, and predicts the impact of various influences, especially interventions, on final endpoints (from survival to satisfaction with care) that matter to decision makers (from patients to society), with special emphasis on the use of patient reported outcomes.

Patient friendliness Also known as acceptability. The extent to which the instrument minimizes patient burden with respect to time, comprehension, and sensitive topics.

Patient reported outcomes (PRO) An instrument that patients complete by themselves or, when necessary, others on their behalf to obtain information in relation to functional ability, symptoms, health status, health-related quality of life, and results on specific treatment strategies. PRO measures can be generic (attempting to assess the consequences of an injury/ disease on the overall well being of a patient), or disease/site-specific (attempting to assess the consequences of a disease or injury of a specific anatomic site on certain behaviors associated with that disease or injury).

Physiologic outcome measures Measures usually assessed by an individual other than the patient and include radiographic measurements such as alignment and union, range of joint motion, muscular strength, and laboratory findings. These measures are usually considered "objective" measurements and are often surrogate measures for other outcomes. They often lack validity and reliability testing.

Population The group of patients tested in the study and described in terms of the condition (disease, injury or surgical intervention), age, and sex.

Reliability The ability of a measure to produce the same results with repeat assessment by the same observer (intra-observer reliability) or by different observers (inter-observer reliability).

Reproducibility A form of reliability that can be further subdivided into: *inter-observer* and *test-retest*. How closely one observer agrees with another observer using the same instrument and the same patient is the essence of *inter-observer reproducibility*. This form of reproducibility is applicable to clinician based outcomes. *Test-retest reproducibility* is measured by administering the same instrument to the same patient on two different occasions when no important dimensions of health have changed.

Responsiveness Also known as sensitivity to change. It is the ability of a measure to detect a change when a change has occurred. In particular, it measures how well an instrument can detect changes in response to some intervention

Validity The ability of the measure to assess accurately what it purports to assess.

11 List of assessed instruments

A

B

C

D

E

F

G

H

I

K

L

M

N

O

P

Q

R

S

T

U

V

W